Case Studies in Abdominal and Pelvic Imaging

Rita Joarder • Neil Crundwell
Matthew Gibson

Case Studies
in Abdominal
and Pelvic Imaging

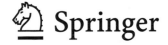 Springer

Authors
Rita Joarder, BSc., MBBS, FRCP, FRCR
Conquest Hospital
St. Leonards-on-Sea
East Sussex
UK

Matthew Gibson, BMedSci, BM BS,
MRCP, FRCR
Royal Berkshire Hospital
Reading
UK

Neil Crundwell, MRCP, FRCR
Conquest Hospital
St. Leonards-on-Sea
East Sussex
UK

ISBN 978-0-85729-365-7   e-ISBN 978-0-85729-366-4
DOI 10.1007/978-0-85729-366-4
Springer London Dordrecht Heidelberg New York

A catalogue record for this book is available from the British Library

Library of Congress Control Number: 2011922532

Cover design: eStudioCalamar, Figueres/Berlin

Printed on acid-free paper

Springer is part of Springer Science+Business Media (www.springer.com)

To Martin, Alfred, Arnold and Freddie, for making it all worthwhile. Thanks also to my parents Robin and Gisela Joarder for all their support over the years.

Rita Joarder

Dedicated to my wife and children for being themselves and all anyone could ask for. Thanks to my generous colleagues in Reading who selflessly contributed some of the cases.

Matthew Gibson

To Kay, Ruth and Mark and in memory of Edwin.

Neil Crundwell

Preface

Case Studies in Abdominal and Pelvic Imaging is a collection of 100 real cases, encompassing a broad range from common medical and surgical problems to more rare but interesting pathologies.

The cases demonstrate the use of modern imaging techniques that are generally commonplace to most hospitals, and illustrate how multiple modalities can be used in the investigation of pathology.

The advent of PACS has meant images are more readily available to clinicians for review in clinics, wards, etc. With the increasing number of multi-disciplinary meetings, the imaging of more cases is reviewed and demonstrated by radiologists to a wider group of clinicians. It is therefore important to have an understanding of imaging and not simply to read the report.

In addition more US is being performed as an extension of examination and a good understanding of the appearances and pathologies that may be demonstrated by this clinician-performed US is essential.

This book is aimed at a broad range of specialties including gastroenterology, general and GI surgery, gynaecology and urology and also radiologists in training and medical students.

In addition, we intend its use to extend to those allied professionals who regularly review imaging when treating their patients, e.g. cancer specialist nurses and endoscopists.

The structure of the book is designed to enable the reader to study 100 cases. Each commences with a brief history, accompanied by the relevant images and questions on one page. The answers to the questions are found on the next page, with annotated images demonstrating the salient features. There is then a brief discussion of the condition, key teaching points, references and suggested further reading. This format reflects changes in medical education, where some of the more traditional formats have been replaced by clinical scenarios which often include an element of imaging.

We hope the cases will be interesting as well as educational.

Rita Joarder
Neil Crundwell
Matthew Gibson

Contents

Abbreviations

AAA	Aortic aneurysm
AD	Autosomal dominant
AFP	Alpha-fetoprotein
AIDS	Acquired immune deficiency syndrome
APCKD	Adult polycystic kidney disease
AXR	Abdominal X-ray
BP	Blood pressure
CA	Coeliac axis
CBD	Common bile duct
CE	Contrast enhanced
CEA	Carcinoembryonic antigen
CEUS	Contrast enhanced ultrasound
CHD	Common hepatic duct
CLO	Campylobacter-like organism test
CRP	C-Reactive protein
CT	Computed tomography
CTA	CT angiogram
CTU	Ct urography, Ct urogram
CXR	Chest X-ray
DWI	Diffusion weighted imaging
ERCP	Endoscopic retrograde cholangiopancreatography
ESR	Erythrocyte sedimentation rate
EUS	Endoscopic ultrasound
EVAR	Endovascular repair
FDG	Fluorine 18 labelled deoxy-glucose
FNA	Fine needle aspiration
FNH	Focal nodular hyperplasia
Gadolinium	
BOPTA	Gadolinium benzyloxypropionictetra-acetate
GB	Gall bladder
GI	Gastro-intestinal
GIST	Gastro intestinal stromal tumour
GP	General Practitioner
GU	Genitourinary tract
Hb	Haemoglobin
HCC	Hepatocellular carcinoma
HRCT	High resolution CT

HU	Houndsfield units
IMA	Inferior mesenteric artery
IMV	Inferior mesenteric vein
IPMT	Intraductal papillary mucinous tumour
IR	Interventional radiology
IV	Intra venous
IVC	Inferior vena cava
IVU	Intra venous urogram
KUB	Kidney Ureters Bladder
LFTs	Liver function tests
MALT	Mucosa-associated lymphoid tissue
MDCT	Multi-detector CT
MIP	Maximum intensity projection
MPR	Multiplanar reformat
MR	Magnetic resonance
MRA	Magnetic resonance angiography
MRCP	Magnetic resonance cholangio pancreatogram
MRF	Mesorectal fascia
MRI	Magnetic resonance imaging
NHL	Non-Hodgkin's lymphoma
OGD	Oesophago gastric duodenoscopy
PCLD	Polycystic liver disease
PDT	Photodynamic therapy
PET	Positron emission tomography
PSA	Prostate specific antigen
PSC	Primary sclerosing cholangitis
PTLD	Post transplantation lymphoproliferative disorder
RIF	Right iliac fossa
RMI	Risk of malignancy index
RT	Renal tumors
RUQ	Right upper quadrant
SBO	Small bowel obstruction
SM	Sclerosing mesenteritis
SMA	Superior mesenteric artery
SMV	Superior mesenteric vein
TAE	Transcatheter arterial embolisation
TCC	Transitional cell carcinoma
TCE	Transcatheter embolisation
UC	Ulcerative colitis
US	Ultrasound
VC	virtual colonoscopy
VUJ	Vesico-ureteric junction
WBC	White blood cell

Case 1

A 78-year-old male with no prior abdominal surgery presented with acute central abdominal pain and vomiting. On examination the abdomen was distended and tympanic with hyperactive bowel sounds. No hernias were palpable. Abdominal x-ray showed dilated small bowel consistent with a distal small bowel obstruction, but cause was not demonstrated.

An MDCT of the abdomen and pelvis was performed (Image 1: Axial of upper abdomen, Image 2: Axial of upper abdomen – just inferior to Image 1 and Image 3: Axial of lower abdomen).

Questions

1. What is arrowed on Image 1? What is this sign called?
2. What are the two organs arrowed on Image 2?
3. What is arrowed on Image 3? Comment on the small bowel in Image 3.
4. What is the diagnosis?

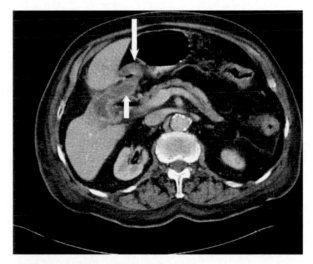

Image 2

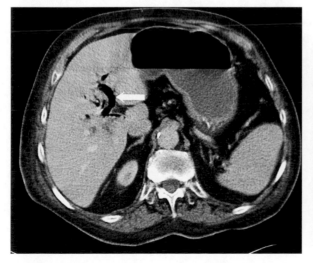

Image 1

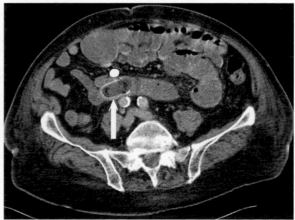

Image 3

R. Joarder et al., *Case Studies in Abdominal and Pelvic Imaging*,
DOI: 10.1007/978-0-85729-366-4_1, © Springer-Verlag London Limited 2011

Answers

1. Air in the intrahepatic bile ducts (*arrow* Image 4) – Aerobilia.
2. The gallbladder (*short arrow* Image 5) and duodenum (*long arrow* Image 3) lying closely adjacent with a bubble air (*long arrowhead* Image 5) between them.
3. A gallstone in the ileum (*long arrow* Image 6) – it has a high density rim with low density material and air within centre of the gallstone. The small bowel proximal to the gallstone is dilated (*medium arrow*) and distal to it is collapsed (*short arrow*), i.e. the gallstone is at the point of transition and the cause of the small bowel obstruction.
4. Gallstone ileus.

Gallstone ileus is a rare complication of gallstone disease, accounting for 1–4% of all bowel obstructions.

Erosion of a gallstone from the gallbladder to the duodenum causes a biliary–enteric fistula. Cholecystoenteric fistulae occur in less than 1% of patients with gallstones. The gallstone passes through the small bowel and may become impacted causing small bowel obstruction. It is most commonly impacted in the distal ileum but can occur anywhere. An exploratory laparotomy with enterolithotomy is indicated. Enterolithotomy is the most commonly used surgical technique with enterolithotomy combined with cholecystectomy and fistulectomy reserved for selected cases. The clinical presentation depends on impaction site and generally includes abdominal pain, nausea and vomiting. Abdominal x-rays may show the aerobilia, dilated small bowel and sometimes the gallstone; however MDCT is more sensitive and thus the imaging of choice.

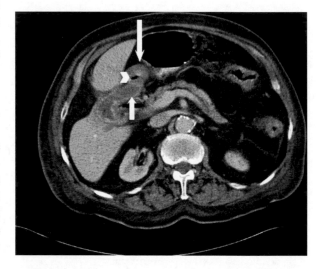

Image 5

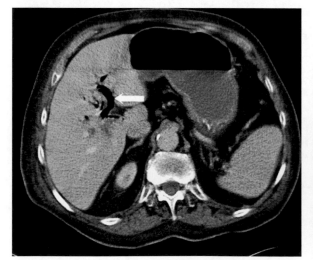

Image 4

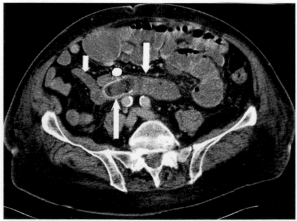

Image 6

Key Points

> Gallstone ileus is an uncommon cause of small bowel obstruction.

> Whilst abdominal x-ray may give the diagnosis CT is usually diagnostic.

Further Readings

Ayantunde AA, Agrawal A. (2007) Gallstone ileus: diagnosis and management. World J Surg 31:1292-7

Muthukumarasamy G, Venkata SP, Shaikh IA, et al. (2008) Gallstone ileus: surgical strategies and clinical outcome. J Dig Dis 9:156-61

A 70 year-old-female with a false eye complained of right upper quadrant pain. She underwent an US of her upper abdomen (Image 1). An MDCT was then performed (Image 2); this was followed by an MRI of which the axial T1 fat sat and T1 sequences are shown (Images 3a and b).

Questions

1. What are the findings on US?
2. What does the MDCT show?
3. What do the unenhanced T1 fat sat and T1 MR sequences show, and what is their significance?
4. What is the likely diagnosis?
5. What further sequences would you perform to clarify appearances?

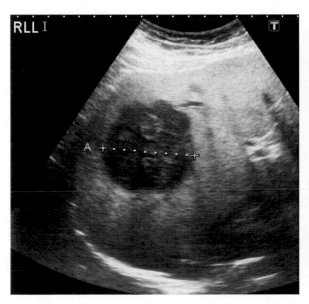

Image 1

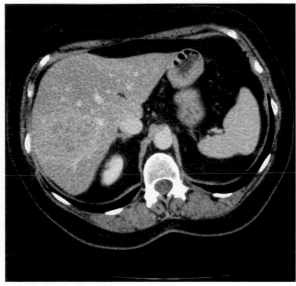

Image 2

R. Joarder et al., *Case Studies in Abdominal and Pelvic Imaging*,
DOI: 10.1007/978-0-85729-366-4_2, © Springer-Verlag London Limited 2011

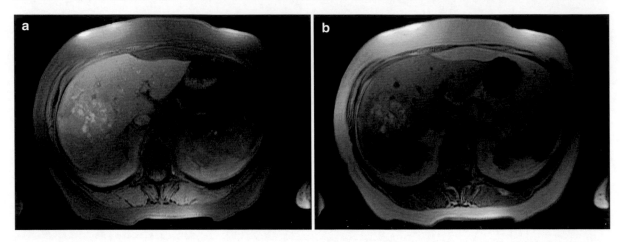

Image 3

Answers

1. The US shows a solitary 5.8 cm solid soft tissue mass within the right lobe of the liver highly suspicious for a metastasis or primary hepatoma (Image 4).
2. The CT confirms a subtle mass within the right lobe of the liver causing distortion of the adjacent vessels (Image 5).

3. MRI (often more sensitive than USS) confirms a 6.8 cm mass that is mixed but predominantly high signal on T1 fat sat imaging (Image 6a) and again mixed signal on T1 with focal areas of high signal within it (Image 6b). The areas of high signal on unenhanced T1 fat sat and T1 imaging indicate either haemorrhage or melanin.
4. The patient had a false eye which would fit with a history of choroidal melanoma, and this is therefore most likely to represent a solitary melanoma metastasis.
5. Dynamic post-gadolinium fat sat T1 scans.

Dynamic post-gadolinium fat sat T1 scans (Images 7a–d) were performed and confirmed arterial enhancement (Image 7a) of the lesion above with wash out of enhancement on portal phase imaging (Image 7b) typical for highly vascular melanoma metastases. Further metastases are revealed only on the

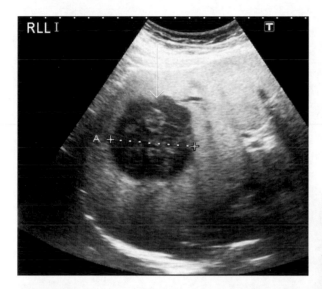

Image 4

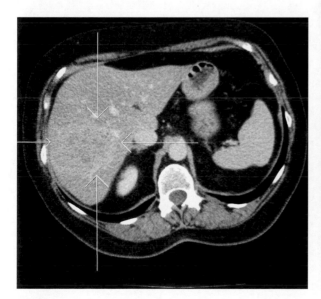

Image 5

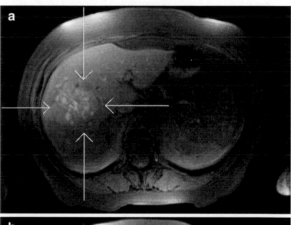

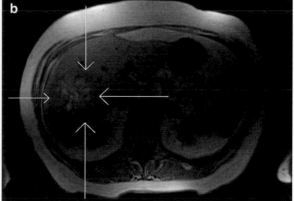

Image 6

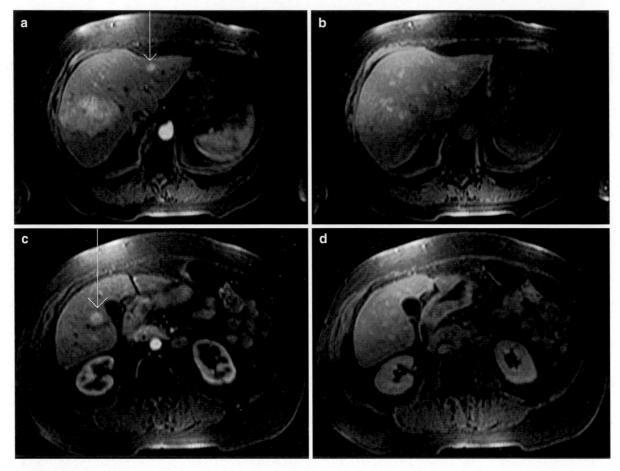

Image 7

post-contrast scan within the left lobe in segments II (*arrow* Image 7a) and V (*arrow* Image 7c) again showing portal phase wash out of enhancement (Images 7b and d).

High signal lesions on T1 imaging include fat, recent haemorrhage, melanin and gadolinium. Highly vascular lesions include hepatomas, neuroendocrine metastases such as carcinoid and renal cell carcinoma metastases. Most other metastases have a portal venous enhancement pattern. Note the significantly increased signal on pre-contrast fat sat T1 imaging which represent areas of melanin.

Choroidal melanoma has a propensity for late hepatic metastases, delays of 10–15 years are not uncommon. This is a different disease pattern to non-choroidal melanoma where spread is most commonly to subcutaneous tissues, lungs and distant lymph nodes. In one series [1] of 25 patients, 15 developed hepatic metastases as the sole initial manifestation of metastatic disease with a median time interval after original enucleation of 43 months and a survival on onset of spread was 7 months.

Key Points

> Choroidal melanoma can metastasize late to the liver.
> Melanin has paramagnetic properties seen as high signal (bright) on T1 and T1 fat sat imaging.
> Differential diagnosis for high signal lesions on T1 imaging are fat, haemorrhage, melanin and gadolinium (on post-contrast scans).
> Other highly vascular lesions include hepatomas, metastases from neuroendocrine tumours such as carcinoid and also renal cell carcinoma metastases.
> MR, particularly with post-gadolinium dynamic scans, greatly increases the sensitivity of hepatic imaging.

Reference

1. Einhorn LH (1974) Metastatic patterns of choroidal melanoma. Cancer 34: 1001-1004

A 70-year-old woman underwent cholecystectomy for symptomatic gall stone disease. Post-operatively she developed a biliary leak, which is managed by endoscopic biliary stenting and external drainage of a gall bladder fossa collection. The external drain dried up but then restarted draining. A CT of the abdomen and pelvis is performed.

Questions

1. What does the CT demonstrate?
2. What needs to be done?
   The patient goes home but presented to the Emergency Department 5 days later with diarrhoea and abdominal pain. A further CT is performed.
3. What does the second CT show?

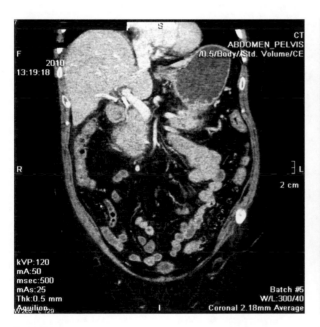

Image 1

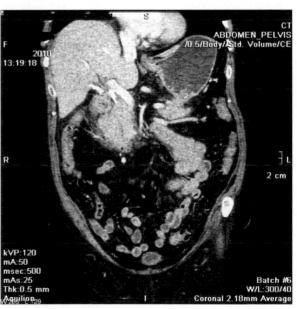

Image 2

R. Joarder et al., *Case Studies in Abdominal and Pelvic Imaging*,
DOI: 10.1007/978-0-85729-366-4_3, © Springer-Verlag London Limited 2011

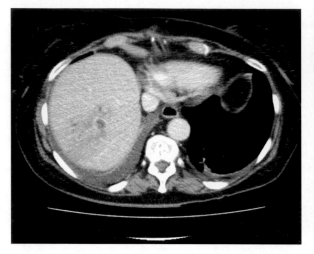

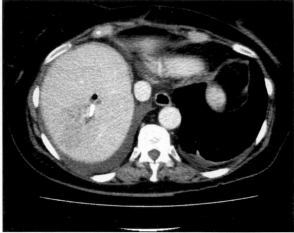

Image 3   **Image 4**

Answers

1. The CT (Image 5) demonstrates the biliary stent (*black arrow*) and the external drain (*white arrow*). The biliary stent has become displaced and its tip lies in the CBD.
2. Repeat ERCP and repositioning of stent or stent replacement is required.
3. The second CT (Image 6) shows high attenuation representing the biliary stent in the high right liver (*black arrow*). There is adjacent very low attenuation in keeping with air (*white arrow*) and some mixed attenuation is seen extending laterally from the tip of the stent. There is fluid attenuation within the lower chest bilaterally in keeping with pleural effusions more on the right.

The mixed attenuation extending from the tip represents a hepatic abscess.

Cholecystectomy is a relative common surgical procedure regarded by some as a minor procedure. Complications include post-operative biliary leak in 0.3–2.7% and stone retention.

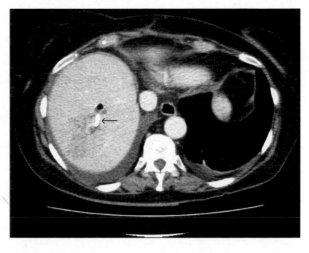

Image 6

Endoscopic intervention is generally accepted as the best treatment for post-operative biliary leak. Complications include ascending infection, stent blockage and migration. Stent migration leads to failure of biliary drainage and there are reported cases of bowel perforation.

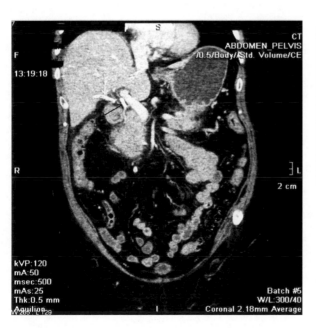

Image 5

Key Points

> Biliary leak is an important complication of cholecystectomy.
> Endoscopic stenting is the preferred treatment option.
> Infection, blockage and migration are the commonest complications of stents.

Further Reading

Ahmad F, Saunders RN, Lloyd GM, Lloyd DM, and Robertson GSM. (2007) An Algorithm for the Management of Bile Leak Following Laparoscopic Cholecystectomy. Ann R Coll Surg Engl 89(1): 51–56.

A previously fit and well 50-year-old male presented with several months of abdominal distension. MDCT of the abdomen and pelvis was performed (Images 1–3. Three non-contiguous axial images.)

Questions

1. Describe the material within the peritoneal cavity.
2. Is there any other abnormality and what are its characteristics?
3. What is the diagnosis?

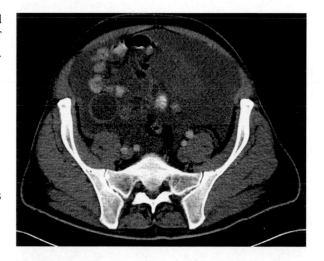

Image 2

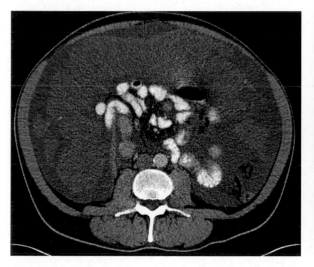

Image 1

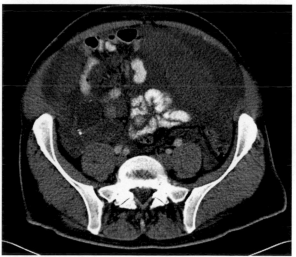

Image 3

R. Joarder et al., *Case Studies in Abdominal and Pelvic Imaging*,
DOI: 10.1007/978-0-85729-366-4_4, © Springer-Verlag London Limited 2011

Answers

1. The CT shows material of two different densities (*long* and *short arrows* Image 4) occupying the peritoneal cavity causing distension of the abdomen with central displacement of bowel.
2. There is a rounded area of low density in the right iliac fossa with subtle mural calcification (*arrows* Images 5 and 6).
3. Pseudomyxoma peritonei due to mucinous adeno-carcinoma of the appendix.

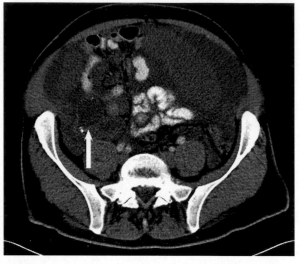

Image 6

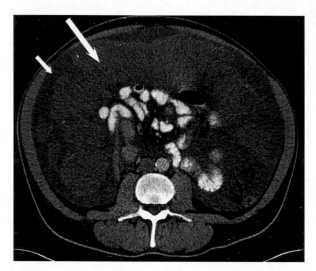

Image 4

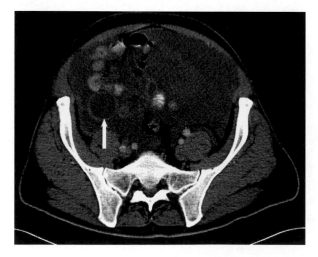

Image 5

Pseudomyxoma peritonei is the clinical syndrome of recurrent mucinous ascites causing abdominal distension. The commonest cause is low-grade mucinous adenocarcinoma of the appendix, which spreads to the peritoneal surfaces without the invasion of adjacent tissues or haematogenous or lymphatic spread. Although the tumour is low grade there is no prospect of cure or long-term survival. Current treatment is focused on cytoreductive surgery and perioperative chemotherapy.

CT often shows large-volume ascites with mixed density material – the denser material is the mucinous ascites. The ascites often fills the abdominal cavity and can extend into the pleural cavity or hernial orifices. There may be peritoneal calcification and septae. There are often pressure effects with scalloping of the liver and spleen and central displacement of bowel. Peritoneal and omental (cake) tissue is seen. Appendiceal masses or cysts (as in this case) representing the primary tumour may be seen.

Key Points

> Pseudomyxoma peritonei is recurrent mucinous ascites causing abdominal distension.
> The commonest cause is low grade mucinous adenocarcinoma of the appendix.
> There is no prospect of cure or long-term survival.

Further Readings

Levy AD, Shaw JC, Sobin LH. (2009) Secondary tumours and tumorlike lesions of the peritoneal cavity: imaging features with pathologic correlation. Radiographics 29(2);347-73

Sulkin TV, O'Neill H, Amin AI, et al. (2002) CT in pseudomyxoma peritonei: a review of 17 cases. Clin Radiol:57(7): 608-13

A 69-year-old male presented with epigastric pain and a 4-day history of vomiting. No haematemesis or malaena. Longstanding history of dyspepsia.

O/E Soft abdomen and mildly distended with epigastric tenderness. An AXR (Image 1) and an US of the upper abdomen (Image 2) were performed.

Questions

1. What does Image 1 show?
2. What does Image 2 show?
3. What is the most likely cause and how would you further investigate this patient?

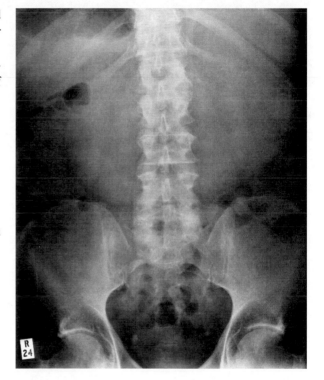

Image 1

R. Joarder et al., *Case Studies in Abdominal and Pelvic Imaging*,
DOI: 10.1007/978-0-85729-366-4_5, © Springer-Verlag London Limited 2011

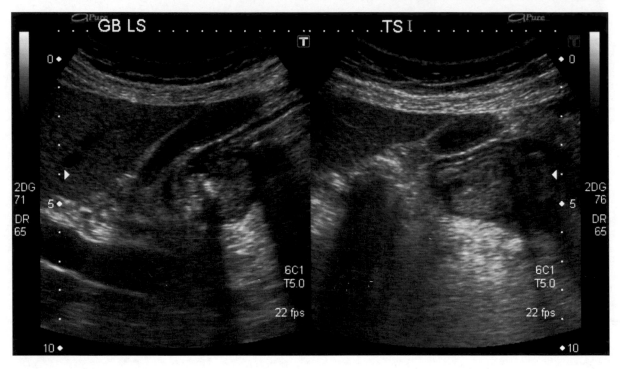

Image 2

Answers

1. A large soft tissue structure filling the epigastrium and left upper quadrant displacing bowel loops (Image 3). The bowel loops themselves are undistended.
2. The image shows a normal undistended gall bladder (*single arrow* Image 4) and a thickened, oedematous pylorus (*double arrow* Image 4) not usually so easily seen at US.
3. Gastric outflow obstruction due to oedematous pylorus most likely secondary to peptic ulcers, best investigated further with endoscopy.

Image 3 shows a fluid filled distended stomach and Image 4 shows an oedematous pylorus and a fluid filled stomach. The endoscopy confirmed two deep ulcers within the pylorus and three further ulcers within the duodenum. Peptic ulcers are not usually investigated with imaging; however, the history may not always be straightforward and initial imaging investigations for epigastric pain may suggest a gastric cause.

Gastric outflow obstruction can arise from several causes, many of which can be suggested by US, e.g. a pancreatic or more rarely a duodenal malignancy, indirectly as in the case above where the USS reveals an oedematous pylorus.

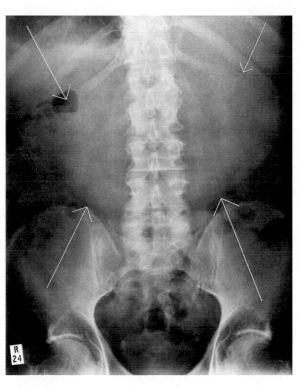

Image 3

Key Points

> US can also exclude other causes of epigastric pain such as acute cholecystitis and hepatic metastases.
> AXR can help to exclude a small bowel obstruction where there is a history of pain, vomiting and abdominal distension.
> Often if no cause is found, CT is helpful in determining the cause.

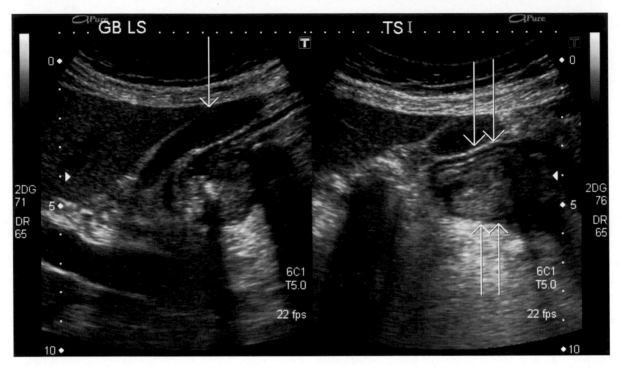

Image 4

A 55-year-old male patient was reviewed on the ward with increasing abdominal pain. He had undergone laparoscopic anterior resection for a rectal polyp at 11 cm from the dentate line. Biopsies had twice shown severe dysplasia.

On examination he was tachycardic and febrile.

A CT scan was requested.

Questions

1. What are the CT findings?
2. What is the diagnosis?

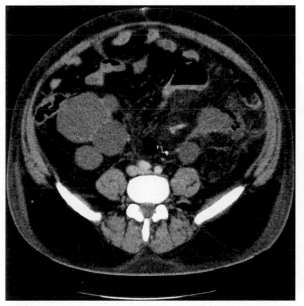

Image 2

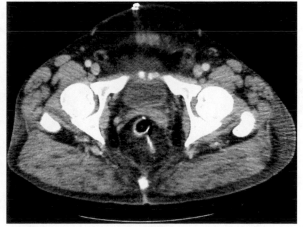

Image 1

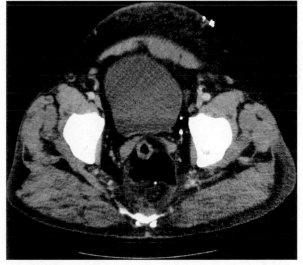

Image 3

R. Joarder et al., *Case Studies in Abdominal and Pelvic Imaging*,
DOI: 10.1007/978-0-85729-366-4_6, © Springer-Verlag London Limited 2011

Answers

1. There is a low attenuation region of free fluid containing air (*short arrow*) in the left iliac fossa (Image 4). The proximal end of the bowel is seen (Image 5). There is high attenuation material representing the suture line (Image 6) in the distal bowel (rectum). The more proximal portion of the bowel is not in continuity with the region of the sutures.
2. There has been dehiscence of the anastomosis.

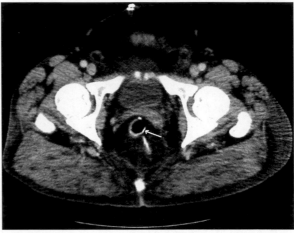

Image 6

The use of laparoscopic surgery is increasing and resections for malignancy or possible malignancy are growing.

Acute complications include conversion to open surgery, anastomotic leak or haemorrhage, with incisional hernia as the most common late complication.

Conversion rates to open operation vary between series with a range from 0% to 8%, as experience with the technique has grown conversion rates have become much lower.

Rates for anastomotic leak vary between 8% and 13.5%. A recent review suggests that complications may be associated with tumour size/site and pathological stage.

Severe dysplasia is part of the spectrum of abnormalities found within adenomatous bowel polyps and is thought to be precancerous. With the advent of mass bowel screening more polyps containing severe dysplasia will be identified. Discussion on an individual patient basis is likely to be required to best plan the options of resection or active follow up.

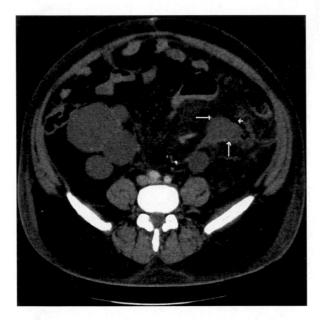

Image 4

> ### Key Points
> › Anastomotic leak is the most common complication of laparoscopic bowel resection.
> › Dehiscence is rare but will lead to an intra-abdominal leak.

Further Reading

Terry M, Neugut A, Bostick R et al (2002) Risk factors for advanced colorectal adenomas: a pooled analysis. Cancer Epidemiol Biomarkers Prev. Jul;11(7):622-9

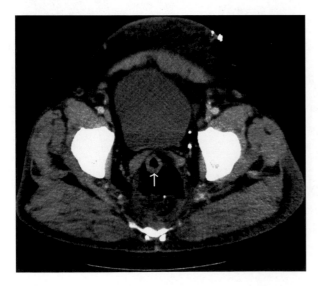

Image 5

A 48-year-old female with a history of carcinoma of the breast underwent US of the abdomen for right upper quadrant pain. A 2-cm hypoechoic solid mass was detected in segment 2 of the liver. MRI of the liver with dynamic contrast enhancement was performed (Image 1 – T1 axial, Image 2 – T2 axial, Image 3 – T1 axial in portal venous phase of dynamic IV gadolinium enhancement).

Questions

1. What is the signal intensity of the lesion on the T1 and T2 weighted images?
2. What is the pattern of contrast enhancement in the portal venous phase?
3. What is the diagnosis?

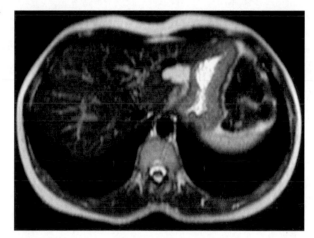

Image 2

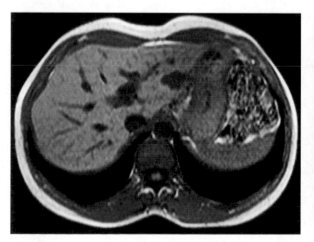

Image 1

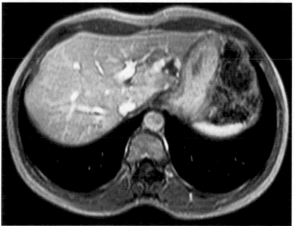

Image 3

R. Joarder et al., *Case Studies in Abdominal and Pelvic Imaging*,
DOI: 10.1007/978-0-85729-366-4_7, © Springer-Verlag London Limited 2011

Answers

1. Low signal on T1 (*arrow* – Image 4) and high signal on T2 (*arrow* – Image 5).
2. Nodular peripheral discontinuus gadolinium enhancement (*arrow* – Image 6).
3. Hepatic haemangioma.

Incidental focal liver lesions are common findings on cross-sectional imaging.

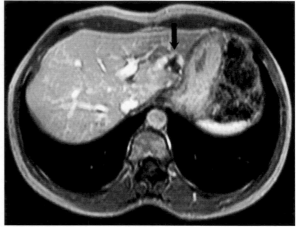

Image 6

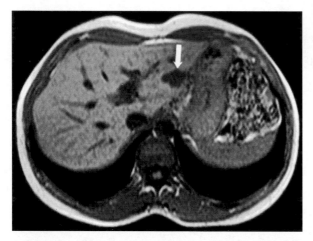

Image 4

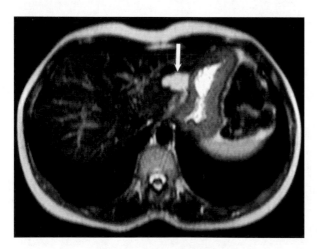

Image 5

Ultrasound is useful to distinguish simple cysts from solid lesions.

If solid, the CT and US appearances can be non-specific and MRI of the liver may clarify.

Hepatic haemangiomas are the commonest benign liver tumour.

On MRI many have a typical appearance. They are usually well defined with low signal on T1 and markedly high signal on T2. Their characteristic peripheral discontinuous nodular pattern of contrast enhancement allows for the firm diagnosis – often obviating further imaging – biopsy or follow-up (very occasionally, some peripheral large lesions may need resection due to the risk of haemorrhage).

Key Points

> Contrast enhanced MRI is useful in evaluating focal hepatic lesions.
> Hepatic haemangiomas often have a typical contrast enhancement pattern allowing confident diagnosis.

A 26-year-old male presented to the Emergency Department with right loin pain and vomiting. Images 1, 2 and 3 are the control, 45 minute and 1 hour and 50 minute films from an IVU.

Questions

1. What does the control film show?
2. What are the possible background diagnoses?
3. What is the cause of the patient's pain?

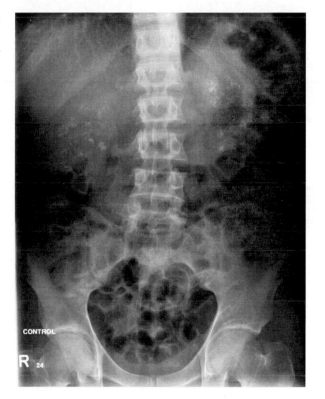

Image 1

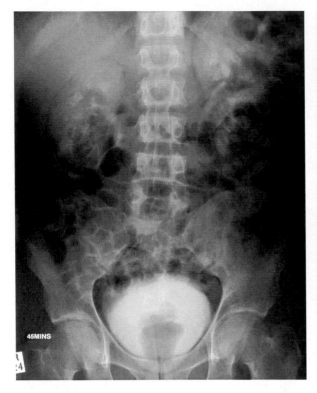

Image 2

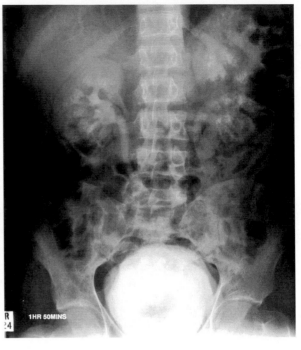

Image 3

Answers

1. Bilateral medullary nephrocalcinosis and three renal calculi within the right pelvicalyceal system (Image 4).
2. There are many causes which include: hyperparathyroidism, renal tubular acidosis, medullary sponge kidney, renal papillary necrosis, any cause of hypercalcaemia or hypercalciuria, and primary hyperoxaluria (rare).
3. The three largest calculi on the right are seen to move in and out of the upper ureter. On the control film there are three calculi within the right renal pelvis (Image 4). On the 45 min film two of the three renal calculi on the right have dropped into the upper ureter (Image 5). On the 1 h 50 min film a 6-mm calculus has dropped down the ureter (Image 6) and is probably causing intermittent obstruction.

Image 6 shows the obstructing calculus. An earlier US (Image 7) shows bright echogenic foci within both kidneys with acoustic shadowing consistent with the dense renal parenchymal calcification.

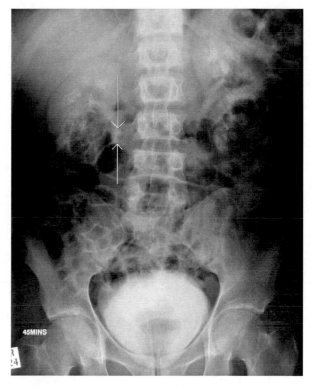

Image 5

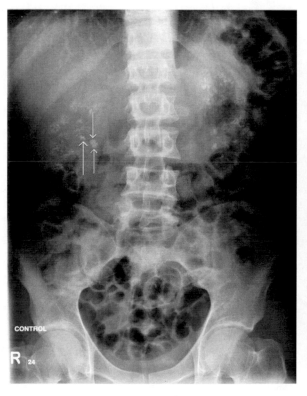

Image 4

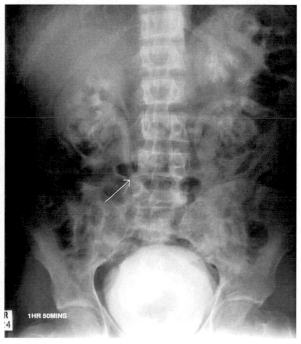

Image 6

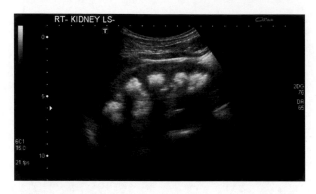

Image 7

Nephrocalcinosis is characterised by the presence of calcium deposits within the renal parenchyma seen on plain film, US and CT. There are two distinct patterns. Medullary, as in this case, with the calcification involving the renal pyramids and cortical.

The patient had renal tubular acidosis diagnosed as an infant, as the cause of medullary nephrocalcinosis; however, there is also a predisposition to developing renal calculi as in this case.

Key Points

> Ninety-five percent of all nephrocalcinosis is medullary (as opposed to cortical).
> There are many causes of medullary nephro-calcinosis listed above.
> Renal calculi can be mobile, even moving in and out of the ureter causing intermittent obstruction.

Further Reading

Rothstein M et al (1990) Renal tubular acidosis. Endocrinol Metab Clin North Am 19(4):869-87

A 54-year-old man presented with rectal bleeding and was found to have a rectal tumour. A staging MRI and CT were arranged.

Questions

1. What does the CT scan show?
2. What is the most likely underlying diagnosis?
3. What is the connection with the rectal tumour?

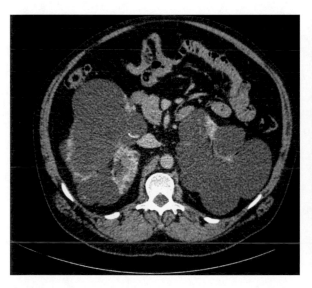

Image 1

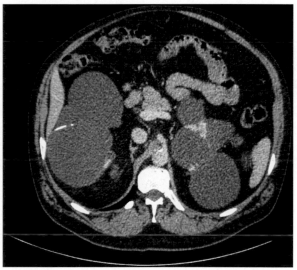

Image 2

R. Joarder et al., *Case Studies in Abdominal and Pelvic Imaging*,
DOI: 10.1007/978-0-85729-366-4_9, © Springer-Verlag London Limited 2011

Answers

1. The CT scan shows multiple low attenuation areas within both kidneys which are almost replacing the renal parenchyma. Some of these contain regions of curvilinear calcific density (Image 3 *arrow*).
2. The CT features are of multiple renal cysts. The most likely diagnosis is of adult polycystic kidney disease (APCKD).
3. There is no association of APCKD with rectal tumours.

APCKD is an inherited abnormality of the kidneys. Inheritance is autosomal dominant.

Individuals may be asymptomatic or may present with flank pain, haematuria, renal colic, urinary tract infections or hypertension. There may be a gradual decline in renal function.

There is an association with cysts in other organs, particularly the liver. There is also an increased incidence of intracranial aneurysms.

Whilst cysts may become septated and contain calcification, there is no link with renal neoplasia.

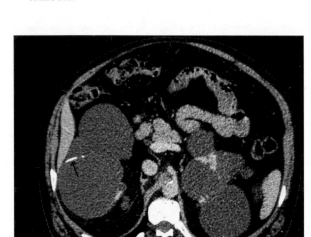

Image 3

Key Points

> APCKD may be asymptomatic, genetic screening is available.
> Intracranial aneurysms are an important association

Further Reading

Torres VE, Harris PC, Pirson Y. (2007) Autosomal dominant polycystic kidney disease. Lancet 369(9569):1287-301

A 67-year-old male patient with alcohol-induced cirrhosis underwent US of the liver and measurement of serum alpha-fetoprotein (AFP) level as part of annual surveillance for hepatocellular carcinoma (HCC).

The AFP level was normal but US revealed two 3-cm lesions in segment 7 of the right lobe of the liver.

An MRI of the liver including both dynamic and hepatobiliary phase contrast enhancement with Gadolinium BOPTA was performed (Image 1, T1 fat saturated axial; Image 2, T2 axial; Image 3, TI axial arterial enhancement; Image 4, T1 axial portal venous enhancement and Image 5, T1 axial hepatobiliary enhancement).

Questions

1. What signal characteristic do the two lesions in the right lobe of the liver show?

2. What are the enhancement patterns in the dynamic and hepatobiliary phases of contrast enhancement?
3. What are the nodules?

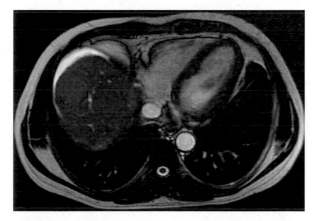

Image 2

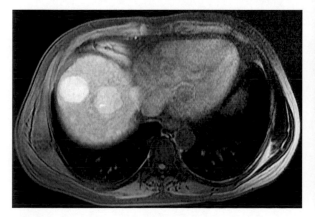

Image 1

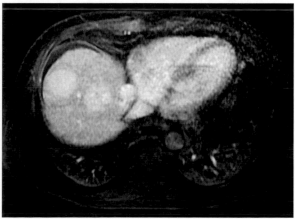

Image 3

R. Joarder et al., *Case Studies in Abdominal and Pelvic Imaging*,
DOI: 10.1007/978-0-85729-366-4_10, © Springer-Verlag London Limited 2011

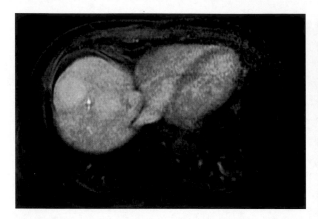

Image 4

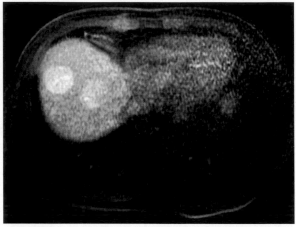

Image 5

Answers

1. High signal on T1 and iso-intense on T2 (*arrows* Images 6 and 7).
2. No abnormal enhancement in dynamic or hepato-biliary phases, i.e. enhances in a similar way to adjacent liver parenchyma (*arrows* Images 8–10).
3. Dysplastic hepatic nodules.

In cirrhosis several sorts of nodules can be seen – including cirrhotic nodules, large regenerative nodules, dysplastic nodules and hepatocellular carcinoma.

The lesions in this case can be confidently diagnosed as dysplastic nodules from their signal characteristic and enhancement pattern. They are typically high signal

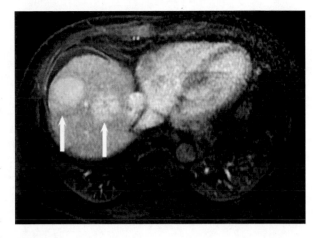

Image 8

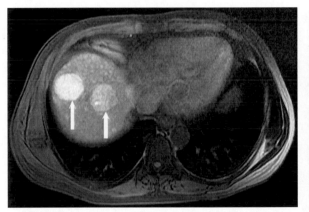

Image 6

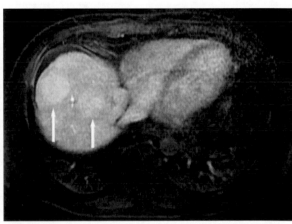

Image 9

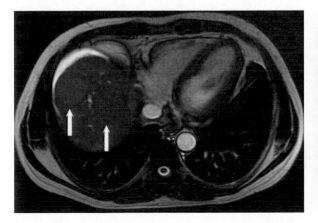

Image 7

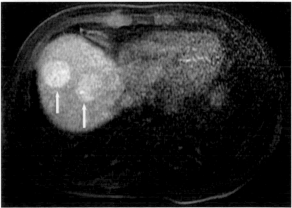

Image 10

on T1, iso-signal on T2 with similar enhancement to "normal" hepatic parenchyma. There is a well-recognised progression from large regenerative nodules through dysplastic nodules to hepatocellular carcinoma.

Key Points

> There are several different types of nodules seen in cirrhosis.
> Unenhanced ultrasound is used for nodule detection.
> Contrast-enhanced MRI is used for nodule characterisation.

Further Readings

Kim MJ, Choi JY, Chung YE, et al. (2008) Magnetic resonance imaging of hepatocellular carcinoma using contrast media. Oncology 75(suppl1):72-82

Kudo M. (2009) Multistep human hepatocarcinogenesis: correlation of imaging with pathology. J Gastroenterol 44(suppl XIX):112-8

Case 11

A 72-year-old male was found on USS to have a 6.3-cm infra-renal aortic aneurysm. He had a 2-year history of treated adenocarcinoma of the prostate. The PSA had reduced from 32 μg/L (at diagnosis) to <0.04 μg/L with Casodex alone and was stable. He was referred to the vascular surgeons who requested an MDCT of his aorta prior to consideration for surgery (Images 1a–c and 2a–c).

Questions

1. What do Images 1a–c show?
2. What does Images 2a–c show?
3. What is the likely diagnosis?

R. Joarder et al., *Case Studies in Abdominal and Pelvic Imaging*,
DOI: 10.1007/978-0-85729-366-4_11, © Springer-Verlag London Limited 2011

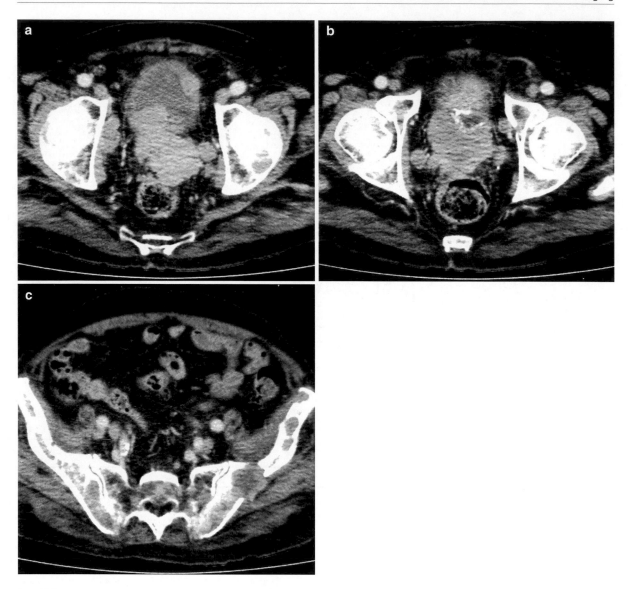

Image 1

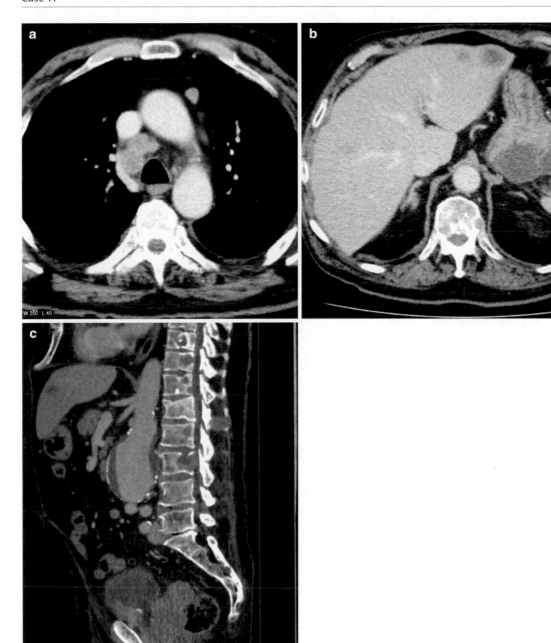

Image 2

Answers

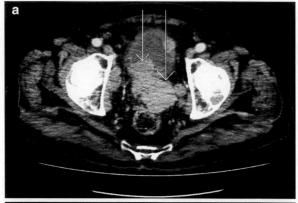

1. CT through the pelvis shows an extensive soft tissue mass arising from the region of the prostate invading the bladder (Image 3a). There is pelvic lymphadenopathy (Image 3b), abnormal focal thickening of the bladder and bony metastases within the pelvis (Image 3c).

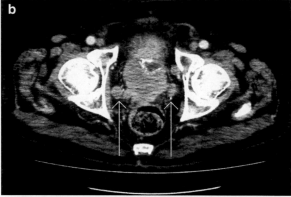

2. CT through the chest shows mediastinal lymphadenopathy within the preaortic and retro-caval regions (Image 4a). The CT through the upper abdomen shows liver metastases (*long arrows* Image 4b) and a peritoneal metastasis invading stomach (*short arrow* Image 4b). The sagittal reconstruction shows the prostatic mass, bladder wall thickening anteriorly, liver metastases, preaortic and mesenteric nodes (Image 4c), abdominal aortic aneurysm and lytic bony metastases involving T10/11/12 and L2/3/4 and 5.
3. Metastatic small cell carcinoma of the prostate.

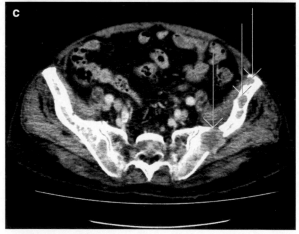

There is extensive metastatic disease and the primary appears to be arising from the prostate. Small cell carcinoma was proven on biopsy. It is unusual for adenocarcinoma of the prostate to be so locally aggressive and to metastasize in this way.

Small cell carcinoma of the prostate is rare but one study found a history of previous usual prostate adenocarcinoma in 42% of patients [1]. The PSA is often normal as in this case. Spread is more likely than with adenocarcinoma most commonly to the bones but also to the lungs and liver.

Image 3

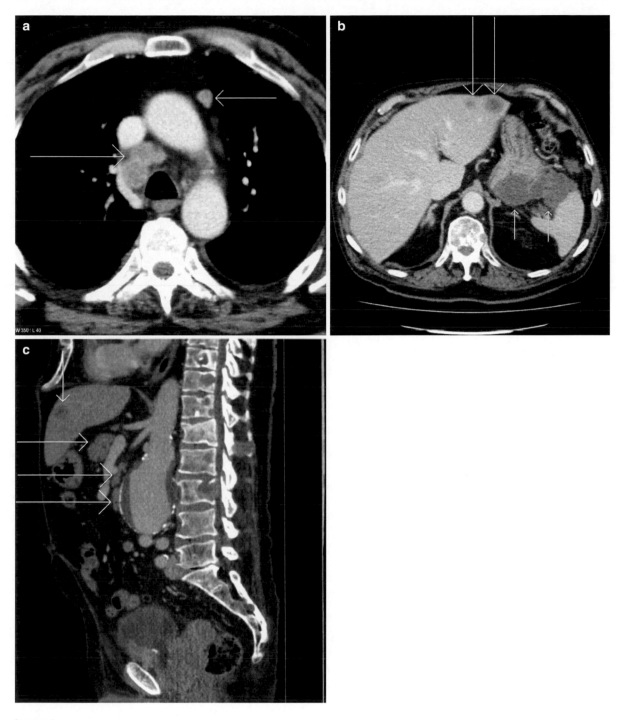

Image 4

Key Points

> Small cell carcinoma of the prostate is rare.
> There is often a previous history of adenocarcinoma of the prostate.
> The PSA can be normal.

Reference

1. Wang W, Epstein JI (2008) Small cell carcinoma of the prostate. A morphologic and immunohistochemical study of 95 cases. Am J Surg Pathol. 32(1):65-71

A 57-year-old woman presented to the Emergency Department with a history of nausea, vomiting and right iliac fossa pain. She had a history of breast cancer treated by mastectomy.

A CT of the abdomen and pelvis is performed.

CT

Questions

1. What abnormalities does the CT scan show?
2. What is the diagnosis?
3. Is there a link with the previous medical history?

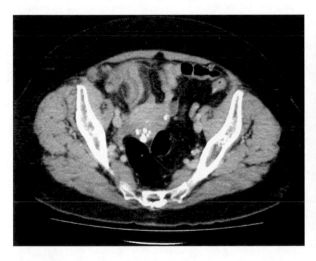

Image 1

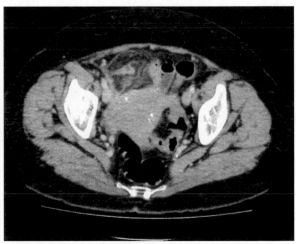

Image 2

R. Joarder et al., *Case Studies in Abdominal and Pelvic Imaging*,
DOI: 10.1007/978-0-85729-366-4_12, © Springer-Verlag London Limited 2011

Answers

1. There is a streaky alteration of attenuation within the mesenteric fat in the pelvis. There is a tubular structure passing around the inferior aspect of the caecal pole (*black arrow*). This is blind ending (Image 3). The wall is thickened with evidence of altered attenuation surround it.
2. The appearances are most suggestive of acute appendicitis.
3. There is no direct link with breast cancer per se. There is an increased incidence of neoplasia in appendectomy specimens in older patients.

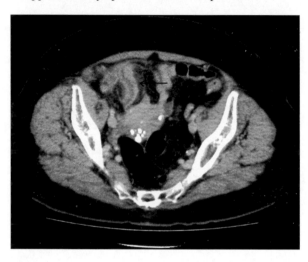

Image 3

Acute appendicitis is a common surgical condition. It more usually presents in younger patients than in this case. With increasing age there is an increasing incidence of malignancy in the resected specimen.

Both US and MDCT are used in the diagnosis of acute appendicitis. There is a preference to use ultrasound first in the paediatric population to avoid ionising radiation. US features are a thickened appendix, local transducer tenderness and peri-appendiceal fat infiltration. On CT appendiceal wall thickening, periappendiceal fat stranding and appendiceal wall enhancement are the most useful findings for diagnosing acute appendicitis. Studies show sensitivity for US or CT of 92% if two features and 96% if three features are present.

> **Key Points**
>
> › Both US and CT can be used in the diagnosis of appendicitis.
> › With increasing age there is an increased incidence of neoplasia.

Further Reading

van Randen A, Lameris W, van Es H et al (2010) Profiles of US and CT imaging features with a high probability of appendicitis. Eur Radiol 20 (7) :1657-66

A 67-year-old male with known cirrhosis secondary to alcohol abuse (who had been abstinent for 8 years) underwent annual liver US and AFP measurement.

After the US was reported as abnormal (Image 1) a contrast enhanced MRI of the liver was performed using Gadolinium BOPTA (Image 2, T1 axial; Image 3, T2 axial; Image 4, arterial phase; Image 5, portal venous phase; Image 6, equilibrium phase of dynamic contrast enhancement; and Image 7, delayed hepato-biliary phase of contrast enhancement)

Questions

1. Describe the ultrasound findings.
2. What diagnosis should be considered?
3. Describe the MRI findings – Signal and enhancement characteristics.

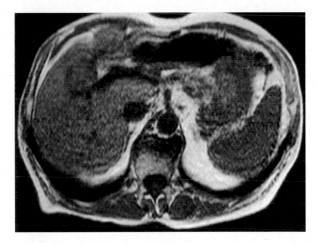

Image 2

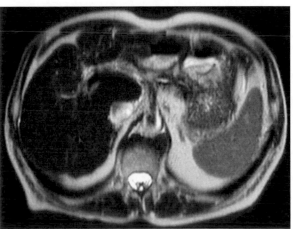

Image 1

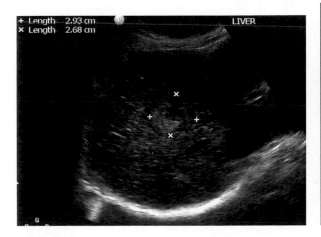

Image 3

R. Joarder et al., *Case Studies in Abdominal and Pelvic Imaging*,
DOI: 10.1007/978-0-85729-366-4_13, © Springer-Verlag London Limited 2011

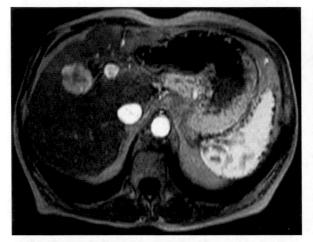

Image 4

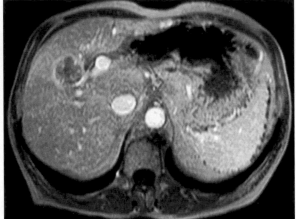

Image 6

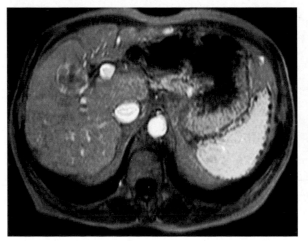

Image 5

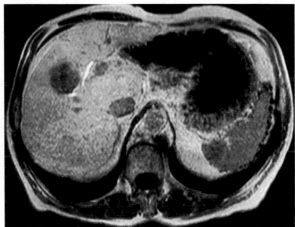

Image 7

Answers

1. 3-cm heterogeneous mass with hypoechoic rim in the centre of the liver (*arrow* Image 8).
2. Hepatocellular carcinoma.
3. 3-cm mass in segment 5 of the liver. Low signal on T1 (*arrow* Image 9), mildly high signal on T2 (*arrow* Image 10). Marked central enhancement in the arterial phase with rapid washout in portal venous and equilibrium phase (*long arrows* Images 11–13). The rim of the lesion is low signal in the arterial phase but enhances in the portal venous and equilibrium phases. No enhancement in the hepatobiliary phase (*arrow* Image 14).

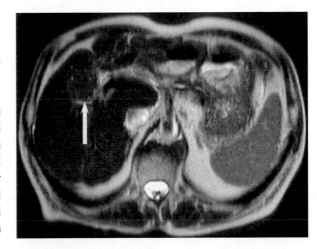

Image 10

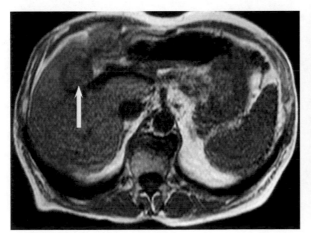

Image 8

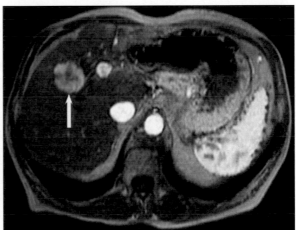

Image 11

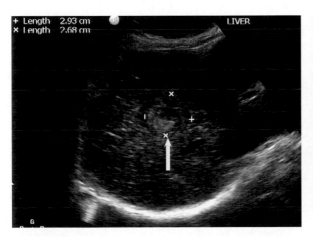

Image 9

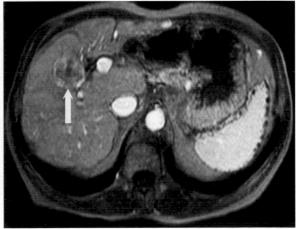

Image 12

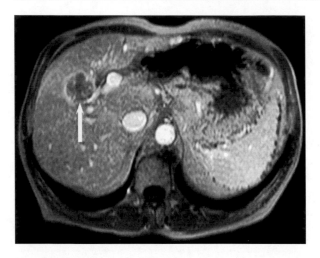

Image 13

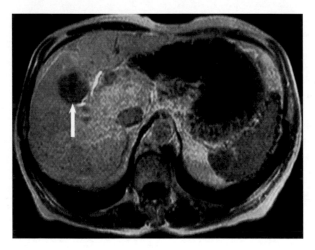

Image 14

Patients at risk of hepatocellular carcinoma are usually monitored with 6-monthly liver US and alpha fetoprotein (AFP).

In this case a solid focal mass lesion was seen on ultrasound. The AFP was normal (it may be in up to 40% of HCCs). MRI was performed for further assessment and this demonstrated the typical signal and enhancement characteristics of HCC.

HCC is usually fairly subtle on the unenhanced sequences. On dynamic enhancement it often shows marked arterial enhancement with rapid washout. The delayed enhancement of the rim reflects a tumour capsule, which is associated with a better prognosis than those tumours without a capsule.

This patient was treated with liver transplantation and the diagnosis confirmed on the extirpated liver.

Key Points

> Patients with cirrhosis should be on an HCC surveillance programme.
> Surveillance is usually with US and AFP.
> MRI is useful for investigating focal abnormalities/nodules detected on US.

A 64-year-old man admitted under the general surgeons with vomiting and abdominal pain. His WBC was minimally raised and his ESR was 74. An AXR (Image 1) and a CT of the abdomen and pelvis (Images 2a, b and 3) were performed.

Questions

1. What does Image 1 show?
2. What do Images 2a and b show?
3. What does Image 3 show?
4. What are the diagnoses?

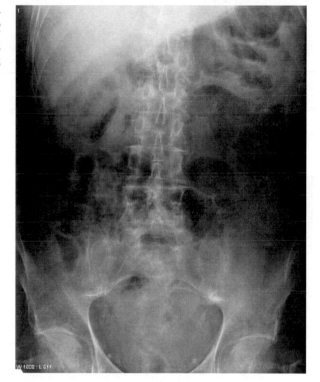

Image 1

R. Joarder et al., *Case Studies in Abdominal and Pelvic Imaging*,
DOI: 10.1007/978-0-85729-366-4_14, © Springer-Verlag London Limited 2011

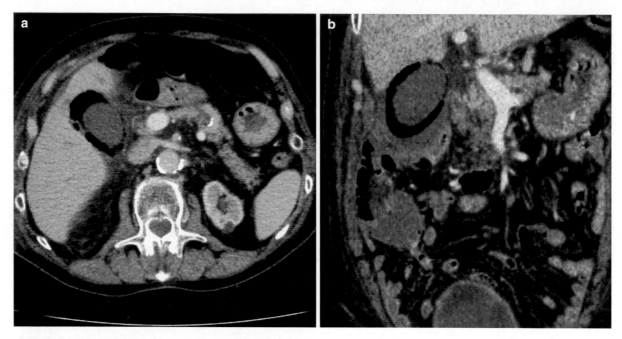

Image 2

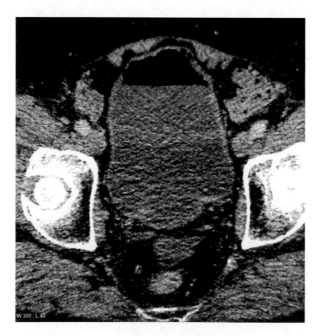

Image 3

Answers

1. The AXR shows a 10 × 6 cm oval partly air attenu-ation mass in the right upper quadrant (*circle* Image 4). Some minor distension of small bowel loops in the left upper quadrant.
2. The axial (Image 5a) and coronal (Image 5b) CT through the upper abdomen shows air in the wall of the gall bladder.
3. The axial CT through the pelvis shows air within the bladder and within the wall of the bladder (*arrows* Image 6).
4. Emphysematous cholecystitis and emphysematous cystitis.

Emphysematous cholecystitis is a rare acute infection of the gallbladder caused by gas forming organisms. The organisms are usually *Escherichia coli*, *Klebsiella* species and less frequently enterococci and anaerobic streptococci. There is felt to be an association with vascular compromise of the gallbladder (and therefore patients with diabetes with small vessel disease), gall-stones and impaired immunity. None of these were the case with the above patient. *E. coli* was grown from blood cultures and urine samples.

Emphysematous cystitis, as seen in this case, is also uncommon and caused by gas forming organisms, most commonly *E. coli*. There is also an association with diabetes and impaired immunity.

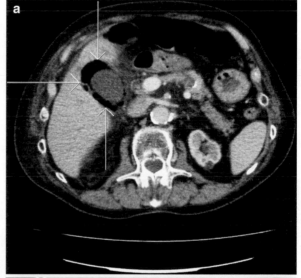
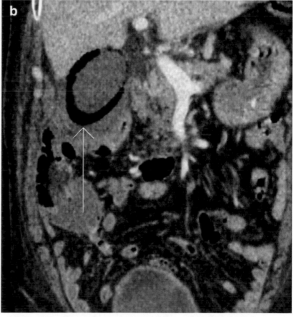

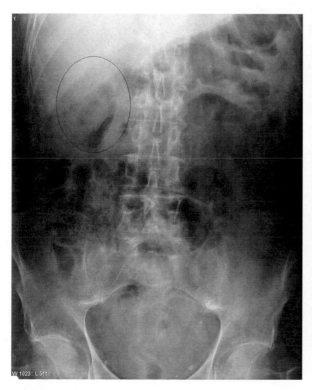

Image 4

Image 5

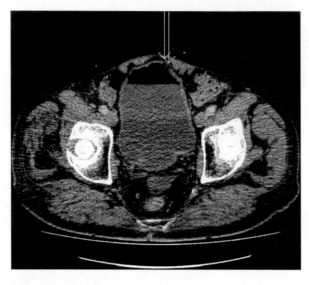

Image 6

Key Points

> Gas forming organisms, most commonly *E. coli*, can cause emphysematous cholecystitis and cystitis.
> Patients with diabetes have a predisposition.

Further Readings

Gill KS et al (1997) The changing face of emphysematous cholecystitis. The British Journal of Radiology 70: 986-991

Grayson DE et al (2002) Emphysematous infections of the abdomen and pelvis: a pictorial review. Radiographics 22: 543-561

A 64-year-old woman was reviewed in out patients. She was known to have pancreatic cancer and has previously undergone ERCP and endoscopic biliary stent placement. She complained of increasing nausea and was jaundiced.

A CT is performed.

Questions

1. What are the CT findings?
2. What complication of treatment has occurred?
3. What is the further management?

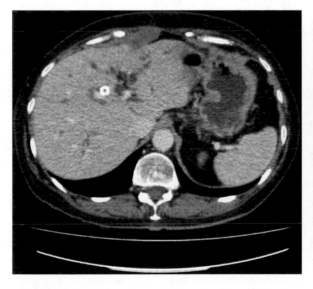

Image 1

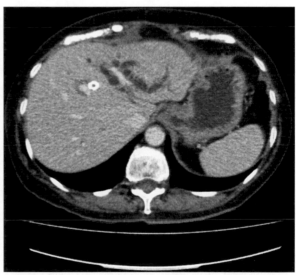

Image 2

R. Joarder et al., *Case Studies in Abdominal and Pelvic Imaging*,
DOI: 10.1007/978-0-85729-366-4_15, © Springer-Verlag London Limited 2011

Answers

1. The CT shows a high attenuation round area in the middle of the liver in keeping with a biliary stent (Image 3 *black arrow*). The intra-hepatic biliary system is demonstrated by the relative low attenuation curvilinear regions. There is dilatation particularly on the left (*white arrow*). There is no evidence of intra-biliary free air.
2. The biliary system is not draining. This may be as a result of stent blockage or displacement.
3. Assessment via endoscopic retrograde cholangiopancreatography (ERCP) is required with stent replacement or repositioning. If ERCP is not possible or fails image guided percutaneous transhepatic intervention may be necessary.

Gas within the biliary system most commonly results from sphincter of Oddi incompetence. This may be post-sphincterotomy or the passage of a gall stone or post-biliary stenting. It may also occur in gall stone ileus (fistulous connection between biliary system and (usually small) bowel, post-trauma, post-operatively, e.g. choleystoenterostomy and as a complication of duodenal ulceration with fistula formation to the common bile duct.

Gas in the biliary system may persist for some time after the introducing event. Lack of gas within a biliary system that has been stented is an indication of stent failure. The degree of biliary dilation is less reliable. Stenting of a chronically obstructed system does not always result in the radicals return to their 'normal' size.

The benefit of biliary stenting prior to pancreaticoduodenectomy is under debate. Studies have shown that pre-operative biliary drainage is associated with a high incidence of bacterobilia and fungal colonization and that a positive intraoperative bile culture is associated with higher morbidity and mortality rates following pancreaticoduodenectomy. In one study a positive culture in the stented patients was related to stent complications and duration of stenting; however uncomplicated stenting was not associated with increased morbidity or mortality. Some authors feel on review there is insufficient controlled data; although some authors feel pre-operative stenting should not be used routinely.

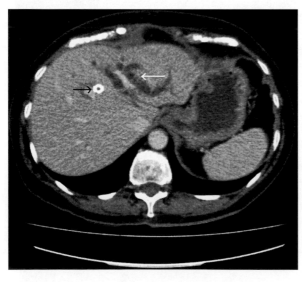

Image 3

Key Points

> Biliary stenting is very useful in the palliative treatment of obstructive jaundice although its role pre-operatively remains uncertain.
> Absence of gas in the biliary system is an indication of stent failure.
> An increase in size of the biliary system post-decompression is also an indication of stent failure. Failure of the biliary tree to reduce in size is not always an indication of a non-functioning stent.

Further Reading

Wang Q, Gurusamy K, Lin H et al (2008) Preoperative biliary drainage for obstructive jaundice. Cochrane Database Syst Rev.16;(3):CD005444

A 65-year-old female, previously fit and well, presented with non-specific abdominal pain and was referred for upper abdominal US. This was abnormal and therefore MRCP was requested (Image 1, T2 axial image of the upper abdomen and Image 2, MIP of the biliary and pancreatic ductal systems).

Questions

1. Describe the findings in Images 1 and 2 – location of abnormality, signal characteristics and relationship to pancreatic duct.
2. What is the differential diagnosis?
3. What would you do next?

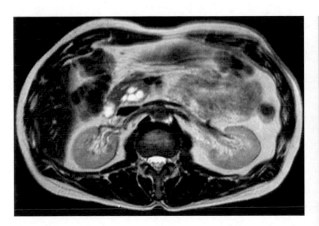

Image 1

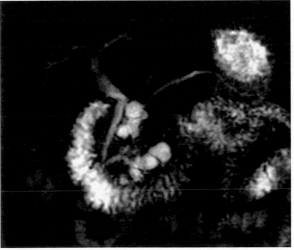

Image 2

R. Joarder et al., *Case Studies in Abdominal and Pelvic Imaging*,
DOI: 10.1007/978-0-85729-366-4_16, © Springer-Verlag London Limited 2011

Answers

1. Well-defined, lobulated areas of T2 high signal in the uncinate process and head of the pancreas (*long arrows* Images 3 and 4) that communicate with the pancreatic ductal system (*short arrows* Image 4).
2. The communication with duct suggests an intraductal papillary mucinous tumour (IPMT). Other diagnoses to consider include other cystic pancreatic tumours, pseudocysts and ductal dilatation due to chronic pancreatitis.
3. If cross-sectional imaging cannot clearly distinguish IPMT from chronic pancreatitis ERCP may be helpful. It can demonstrate communication between the cyst and the duct and sometimes mucin

is seen extruding from the papilla (both suggesting IPMT). However endoscopic ultrasound (EUS) is now the preferred investigation. The relationship to the pancreatic duct is usually well seen. Tumour nodules may be seen and diagnostic aspiration (FNA) of these can be performed. Cyst fluid/mucin and pancreatic juice can be aspirated for cytology, tumour markers and amylase levels.

IPMTs have been recognised since the 1980s and referred to by various names. In 1997 the unifying term intraductal papillary mucinous tumour (IPMT) was adopted.

These tumours arise from the epithelial lining of the pancreatic ductal system, produce mucin and, therefore, cause dilatation of the pancreatic ductal system. They may arise from the main duct or the side branches. Histologically, they range from hyperplasia (premalignant) to carcinoma.

Roughly equal sex distribution and present most often in late middle age.

Often found incidentally on cross-sectional imaging but can present with abdominal pain or pancreatitis. The tumours progress fairly slowly and are slow to metastasise but late in the disease process can cause jaundice, duodenal or gastric compression and peritoneal disease.

US is usually non-specific often demonstrating a cyst in the pancreas but unable to see relationship to the pancreatic duct. CT and MRI/MRCP show pancreatic duct or side branch dilation, which communicate with the cyst (Image 5, different case – axial CT showing a cyst communicating with the pancreatic duct). Pancreatic atrophy is common. If CT or MRI are not diagnostic then ERCP or EUS are performed (as discussed above).

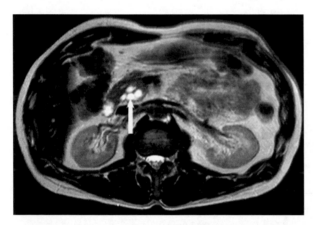

Image 3

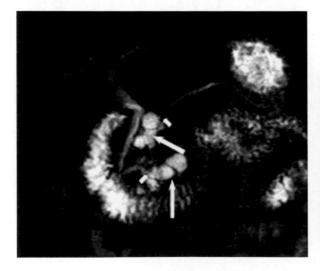

Image 4

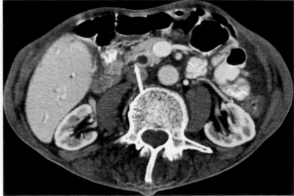

Image 5

Key Points

> IPMT are mucin producing cystic tumours arising from the pancreatic ductal system.
> Histologically IPMTs range from hyperplasia to carcinoma.
> IPMTs are often discovered incidentally and best investigated with EUS.

Further Reading

Procacci C, Megibow AJ, Carbognin G, et al. (1999) Intraductal papillary mucinous tumour of the pancreas; A pictorial essay. Radiographics;19(6):1447-1463

A 74-year-old female with severe Alzheimer's disease and a past history of diverticulitis and Crohn's colitis was admitted from her nursing home with a 1-week history of increasing left leg pain and was unable to stand on admission. An AXR (Image 1) followed by CT of the pelvis (Images 2a–d) were performed.

Questions

1. What is the abnormality on Image 1?
2. What are the abnormalities on Images 2a–d?
3. How does this all fit together?

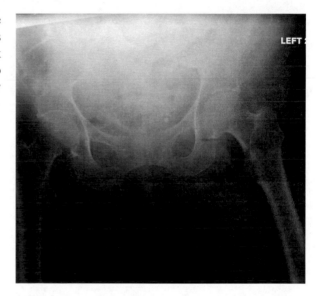

Image 1

R. Joarder et al., *Case Studies in Abdominal and Pelvic Imaging*,
DOI: 10.1007/978-0-85729-366-4_17, © Springer-Verlag London Limited 2011

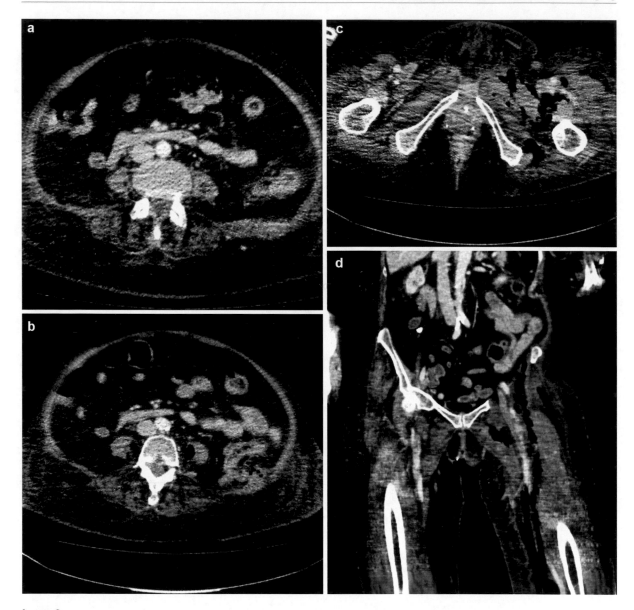

Image 2

Answers

1. Air within the soft tissues around the left hip (Image 3).
2. Image 4a shows thickening of the distal descending colon, Image 4b shows air within the left psoas muscle (*vertical arrow*) and diverticulosis within the descending colon (*horizontal arrows*). Part of the descending colon appears to be adherent to the posterior peritoneum. Images 4c (axial) and d (coronal reconstruction) show air continuous with abnormal descending colon tracking into the left thigh down to the distal femur.
3. The appearances are suggestive of a paracolic abscess resulting from either her past diverticular disease or Crohn's disease. This has formed a fistulous communication with the left psoas and left inguinal region to extend into the soft tissues of the thigh. There was no fluid component to drain.

Fistula formation is a well-recognised complication of both diverticular disease and Crohn's disease. Fistulae can form between bowel and other organs, e.g. colovesical, colovaginal, but can also result in a localised, walled-off perforation or collection. This case is a little unusual in that there is a communication with the psoas muscle and left thigh but no associated abscess within these tissues. Unfortunately, the patient died from the resultant septicaemia.

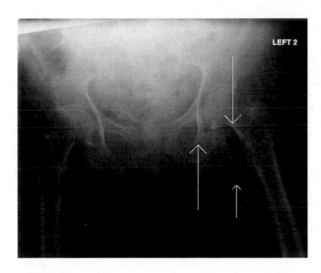

Image 3

Key Points

> Look for abnormalities of the soft tissues even if X-rayed to exclude a fracture.
> A full history, in this case the past medical history, is often helpful.

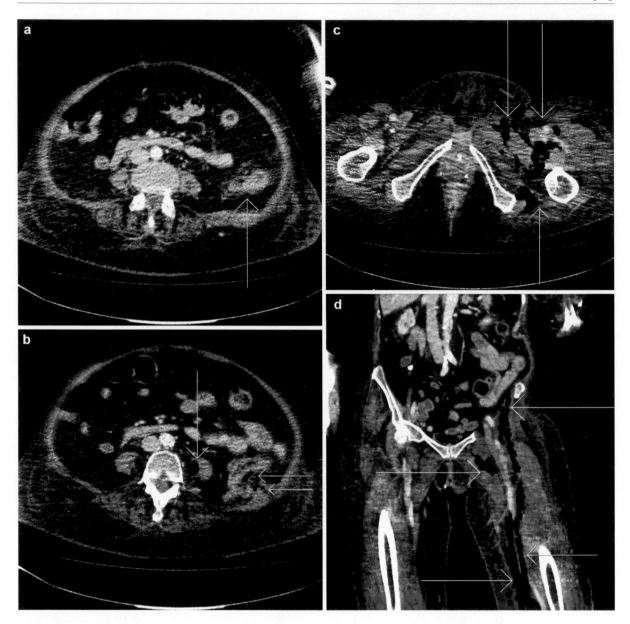

Image 4

A 65-year-old man was investigated for painless haematuria. He had a history of treated stomach cancer.

A CT of the abdomen is performed as part of the
investigation.

Questions

1. What are the CT findings?
2. What is the differential diagnosis for these appearances?

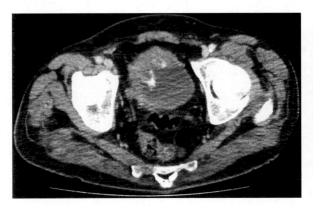

Image 1

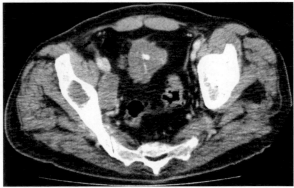

Image 2

R. Joarder et al., *Case Studies in Abdominal and Pelvic Imaging*,
DOI: 10.1007/978-0-85729-366-4_18, © Springer-Verlag London Limited 2011

Answers

1. There is abnormal soft tissue over the anterior lateral wall of the bladder on the right side (Image 4 *white arrow*). This contains very high attenuation consistent with calcification (Image 4 *black arrow*). There is a soft tissue mass in the region of the right iliac vessels measuring some 4 × 2.5 cm consistent with enlarged lymph nodes (Image 5).
2. The features are those of a tumour within the bladder and right iliac chain lymph node enlargement. The bladder tumour may be a primary growth but given the history of malignancy elsewhere a secondary deposit will need to be considered.

The majority of urinary bladder malignancy is primary, with metastatic disease accounting for around 1.5% of malignancies. The most common primaries to metastasise to the bladder are melanoma, stomach, breast, kidney and lung.

Calcification within primary bladder tumours is uncommon, quoted at around 8% although much higher in urachal tumours.

Calcification within metastases has been reported with many primary tumour sites and a range of metastatic locations. Calcification in metastases occurs as a result of two main processes: primary bone formation in tumour osteoid (orthoplastic calcification) or ossification/calcification of tumour cartilage (metaplastic calcification); or secondarily as a result of necrosis, haemorrhage and regressive changes (dystrophic and mucoid calcification). The latter are most commonly seen after radio- or chemotherapy treatment.

Calcification within metastatic disease can mimic calcification within other non-malignant processes such as granuloma formation, parasitic infection and benign neoplasia.

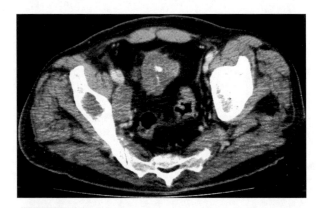

Image 3

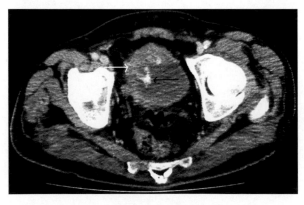

Image 4

Key Points

> Calcification within bladder tumours prior to treatment is uncommon.
> The incidence of calcification within metastatic disease increases with treatment.

Further Reading

Thali-Schwab C, Woodward P, Wagner B(2005) Computed tomographic appearance of urachal adenocarcinomas: review of 25 cases. Eur Radiol. 2005 Jan;15(1):79-84

A 20-year-old male was tackled on his left side during a game of rugby. He presented 12 h later (after celebrations in a nearby hostelry) complaining of pain in the left upper quadrant. On examination he was tender on palpation of the left upper quadrant. Blood pressure, pulse and haemoglobin were normal. There was no haematuria. MDCT of the abdomen and pelvis was performed (Images 1–3 – axials through the upper abdomen).

Questions

1. Describe the findings in the spleen.
2. What is the low attenuation material around the liver?
3. What is the diagnosis?

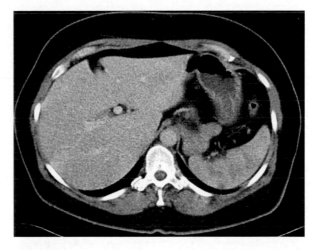

Image 2

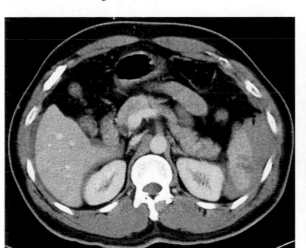

Image 1

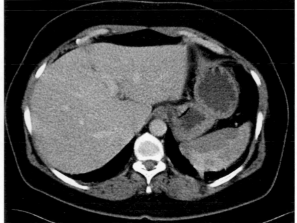

Image 3

R. Joarder et al., *Case Studies in Abdominal and Pelvic Imaging*,
DOI: 10.1007/978-0-85729-366-4_19, © Springer-Verlag London Limited 2011

Answers

1. There are linear tracks of low attenuation (*long arrow* Image 4) passing through the spleen. There is low attenuation around the spleen (*star* Image 4).
2. Perihepatic free fluid (in this case, blood) around the liver (*short arrow* Image 4).
3. Grade 3 splenic laceration with adjacent haematoma and intraperitoneal blood.

CT is the most widely used and accurate way of assessing blunt abdominal injury. Blunt splenic trauma can be graded according to the CT findings. There are several systems, but the most widely used is from the American Association for the Surgery of Trauma [1].

According to this system the case shown has a Grade 3 Injury – the lacerations were greater than 3 cm but did not extend to the hilar vessels or cause devascularisation and there was a 50% subcapsular haematoma, which had ruptured causing intraperitoneal blood.

CT grading systems ensure injuries are described in a standardised fashion and are useful comparing outcomes etc. However, there is controversy about their usefulness in predicting the need for intervention [2].

The management of splenic injuries has gradually changed over recent years. There is a tendency toward conservative management with splenic preservation, if possible (it is often impressive how quickly splenic lacerations heal and are often not visible on follow-up CTs). Intervention may be required for more severe injuries particularly in the context of haemodynamic instability. Operative management has also evolved – the standard is still splenectomy but, if possible, spleen preserving surgery is used. Transcatheter embolization (TCE) in the IR suite is becoming more widespread – there are different techniques but the most widely used is to place metal fibred coils in the main splenic artery (distal to the main supply to the pancreas) to reduce the perfusion pressure in the spleen. Embolization can usually be achieved fairly quickly and usually results in cessation of bleeding; stabilization of the patient and surgery can usually be avoided. However, it requires the rapid response by the Interventional Radiology team.

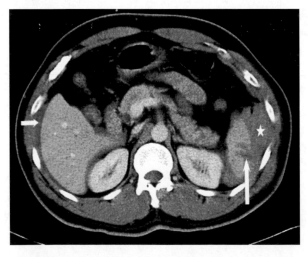

Image 4

Key Points

> Blunt trauma is best imaged by MDCT.
> Splenic injury can be graded by the CT findings.
> TCE is a useful technique for controlling splenic haemorrhage.

References

1. http://www.trauma.org/archive/scores/ois.html
2. Cohn SM, Arango JI, Myers JG, et al. (2009) Computed tomography grading systems poorly predict the need for intervention after splenic and liver injuries. Am Surg 75(2):133-9

An 86-year-old male with a history of worsening renal function and polycythaemia was referred for US (Images 1a and b) of his renal tract. The US prompted a CT of the abdomen and pelvis (Images 2a–d).

Questions

1. What does Images 1a and b show?
2. What does Image 2a show and what is the structure annotated with an *arrow*? Is it normal?
3. What is the abnormal structure annotated with an *arrow* in Image 2b.
4. What do Images 2c and d show and what is the cause of this?

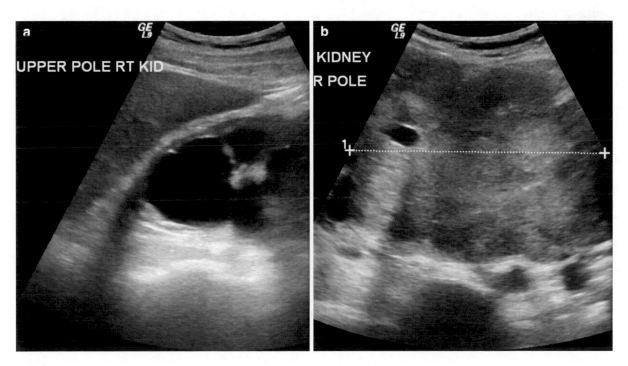

Image 1

R. Joarder et al., *Case Studies in Abdominal and Pelvic Imaging*,
DOI: 10.1007/978-0-85729-366-4_20, © Springer-Verlag London Limited 2011

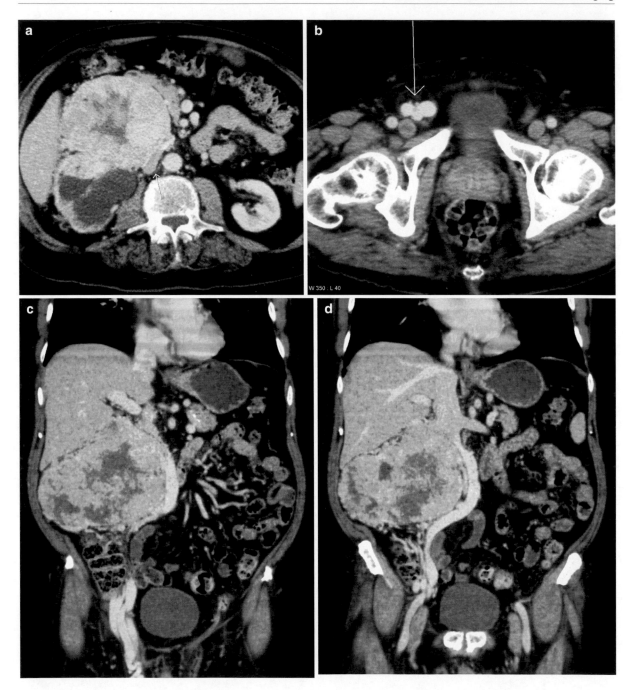

Image 2

Answers

1. A marked hydronephrosis of the upper pole of the right kidney (Image 3a) and a soft tissue mass within the lower pole (Image 3b).
2. The CT shows a large soft tissue mass expanding the right kidney within the mid and lower pole (*vertical arrow* Image 4a) causing obstruction of the more posterior and superior aspect of the collecting system of the rest of the right kidney (*horizontal arrow* Image 4a). The structure annotated with an *arrow* in Image 2b is the IVC, which is significantly compressed. Note the enlarged veins anterior and medial to the renal mass draining the mesentery and bowel.
3. A right sided varicocoele.
4. There is significant dilatation of the right testicular vein (Image 4b) which is seen to drain directly in to

the IVC above the mass (Image 4c). The cause is the compression of the IVC resulting in dilatation of venous collaterals. This also explains the prominent mesenteric veins.

The more usual combination is a left sided renal tumour with involvement of the left renal vein resulting in a left sided varicocoele as the left testicular vein drains into the left renal vein. In this case, the IVC is compressed and so there is retrograde flow up the RT testicular vein into the IVC above the compression.

> ### Key Point
>
> › Whenever a varicocoele is discovered a renal US should be performed.

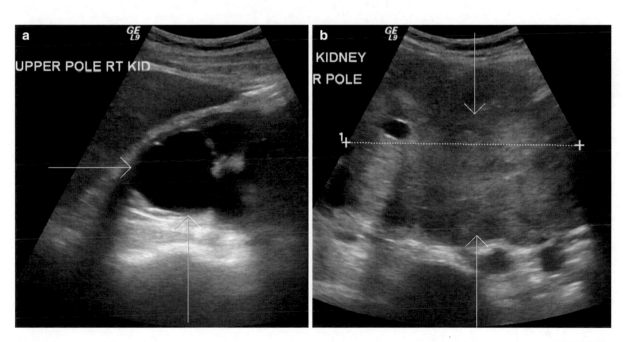

Image 3

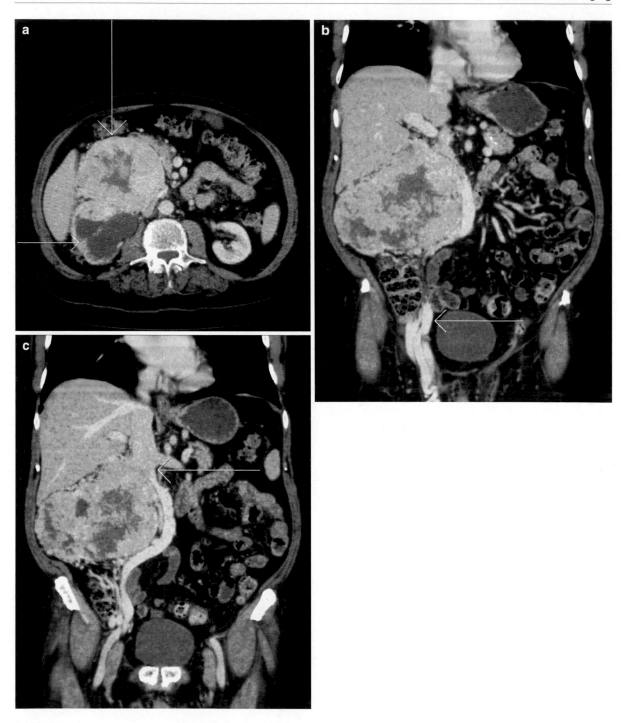

Image 4

Case 21

A 37-year-old female was reviewed in outpatients department. She has a history of Crohn's disease. She had no abdominal pain but commented on very noisy bowels.

An out patient colonoscopy is arranged which fails. Further investigation is requested.

Questions

1. What investigation has been performed?
2. How is it performed?
3. What are the findings?

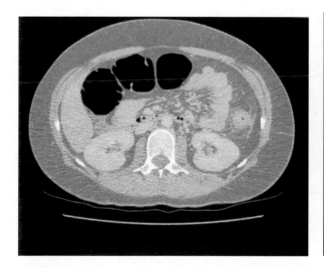

Image 2

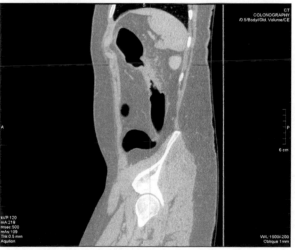

Image 1

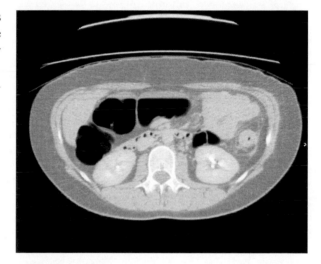

Image 3

R. Joarder et al., *Case Studies in Abdominal and Pelvic Imaging*,
DOI: 10.1007/978-0-85729-366-4_21, © Springer-Verlag London Limited 2011

Answers

1. The investigation is CT colonography (virtual colonoscopy).
2. Bowel preparation is generally as for fibre-optic colonoscopy. After rectal intubation the bowel is distended with either carbon dioxide or air. Images are acquired with the patient supine and prone or in the lateral decubitus position. Imaging may be performed post intravenous contrast and the chest may be included.
3. There is a region of large bowel on the descending colon that is not seen to distend on either supine (Image 4 *black arrow*) or prone (Image 5 *black arrow*) view. This is consistent with a stricture. Given the history of Crohn's disease this is most likely to be inflammatory in origin. Sagittal off-axis reconstruction (Image 6 *white arrow*) allows easy measurement of length.

CT colonography takes advantages of multidetector technology. The data is processed in such a way to not only provide traditional axial, coronal and sagittal reconstructions, but also allow a fly-through view of the bowel, recreating the view at colonoscopy. More recent advances in reconstruction give the ability to produce a 'flattened' sample termed virtual dissection.

Indications for CT colonography include failed or declined colonoscopy and completion staging of an impassable tumour. The techniques role is likely to increase and will almost certainly replace barium enema in the examination of the large bowel. It has the advantage of being generally better tolerated without reduced accuracy, as well as visualising structures outside the bowel.

Advocates suggest that the technique should be used for bowel screening in both symptomatic and asymptomatic patients. Polyps can reliably visualised down to a size of 7 mm. Whilst this has not currently gained acceptance in the UK the technique has recently gained endorsement from US President Obama.

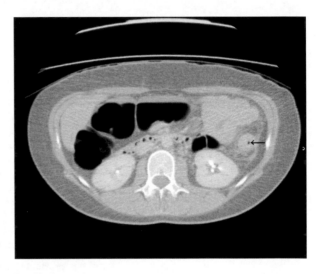

Image 5

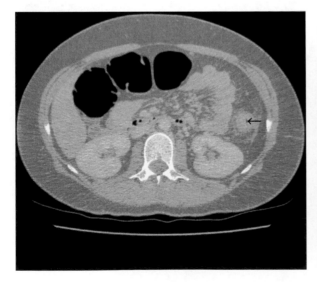

Image 4

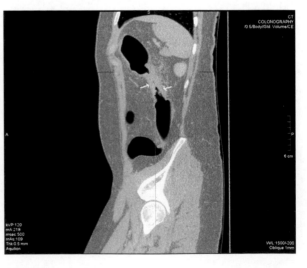

Image 6

Key Points

> Stricture in inflammatory bowel disease may be relatively asymptomatic.

> CT colonography is a technique of increasing importance.

Further Reading

Christensen K, Fidler J, Fletcher J et al (2010) Pictorial review of colonic polyp and mass distortion and recognition with the CT virtual dissection technique. Radiographics 30(5):e42

A 25-year-old male presented with bloody diarrhoea, opening his bowel 15 times per day.

He was tachycardic with generalised abdominal tenderness.

A plain abdominal X-ray (AXR) was performed (Image 1)

Questions

1. Describe the transverse colon.
2. What is the differential diagnosis for this appearance?
3. What is the likely cause in this clinical scenario?
4. What is the semicircular opacity at the bottom of the image (*long arrow* Image 1)?

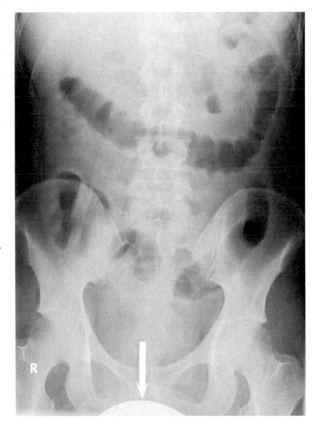

Image 1

R. Joarder et al., *Case Studies in Abdominal and Pelvic Imaging*,
DOI: 10.1007/978-0-85729-366-4_22, © Springer-Verlag London Limited 2011

Answers

1. There is marked thickening of the colonic wall known as "thumb printing" (*short arrows* Image 2) without any bowel dilation.
2. There is a wide differential diagnosis, but two of the most common causes are ischaemic colitis and inflammatory bowel disease.
3. Ulcerative colitis
4. Gonad shield – to protect scrotum from radiation whilst performing AXR – which are often repeated frequently in this scenario (*long arrow* Image 2).

'Thumb printing' is the radiological sign of thickened, oedematous colonic wall. It is classically associated with ischaemic colitis but appears relatively late in the disease process and is associated with a poor prognosis. It is also seen in inflammatory bowel disease – particularly 'toxic megacolon'. Other causes – trauma, infection (amoebic), lymphoma, amyloid and endometriosis – are much less common.

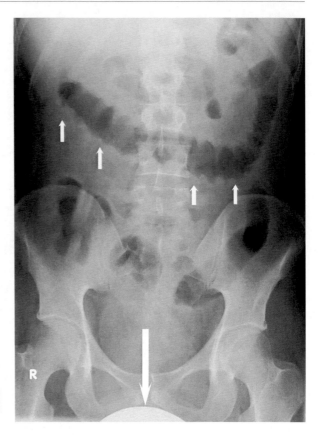

Image 2

Key Points

> Thumb printing is a classical radiological sign on AXR.

> Commonest causes are ischaemic colitis and inflammatory bowel disease.

An 84-year-old male presented with an acute upper GI bleed (Hb 6.8 g/L). An abnormality was seen at endoscopy and endoscopic biopsies taken. An MDCT was performed (Images 1a and b).

Questions

1. What do Images 1a and b show?
2. What is the likely diagnosis?
3. What is the likelihood of malignancy?
4. How do these lesions present?

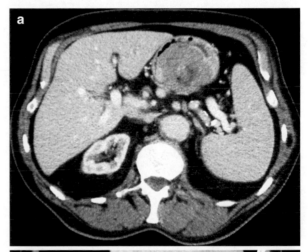
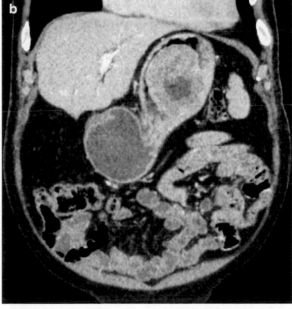

Image 1

R. Joarder et al., *Case Studies in Abdominal and Pelvic Imaging*,
DOI: 10.1007/978-0-85729-366-4_23, © Springer-Verlag London Limited 2011

Answers

1. A well-defined round mass within the fundus of the stomach, inseparable from the stomach wall (Images 2a and b). The mass appears to have a necrotic centre.
2. A gastro-intestinal stromal tumour (GIST).

3. The malignant potential is determined by grade on histology and size of the mass.
4. As in this case, GISTs can bleed. Many, however, are asymptomatic and are incidental findings at OGD or CT.

GISTs are a subset of GI mesenchymal tumours of varying differentiation and originate from the muscularis propria of the intestinal wall. The older medical literature referred to these as leiomyomas or leiomyosarcomas. They are usually found in the stomach but can be found anywhere along the GI tract, the second most common site is the small bowel. Small- and low-grade tumours rarely metastasise; large- and high-grade tumours most commonly metastasise to the liver and peritoneum.

Radiologically they are well-defined round lesions that appear to arise from the stomach or small-bowel wall.

Key Points

> If you see a well-defined mass arising from stomach or small-bowel wall, consider GISTs
> Size matters! Measure lesion accurately.
> Smaller GISTs may be an incidental finding and will require follow up.

Further Reading

Vu H Nguyen, MD et al Gastrointestinal Stromal Tumours - Leiomyoma/Leimyosarcoma: emedicine.medscape.com. article/369803

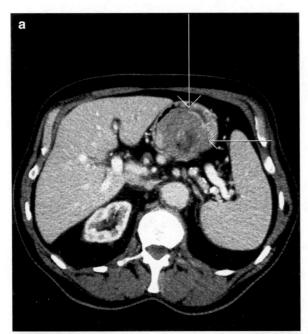

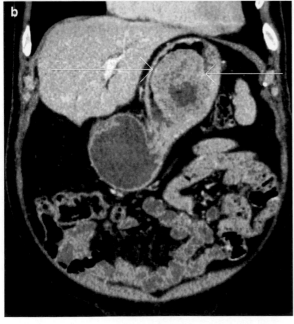

Image 2

An 80-year-old woman was seen in out patients. She had been admitted to hospital with abdominal pain 2 months previously and ultrasound at that time demonstrated a lesion in the bladder. She subsequently underwent transurethral resection of a bladder tumour.

She complained of a change in bowel habit with intermittent upper abdominal pain. Examination was unremarkable. She declined sigmoidoscopy or colonoscopy.

CT colography was requested.

Questions

1. What are the CT findings?
2. What is the diagnosis?
3. What further investigation is required?

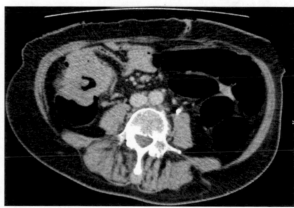

Image 2

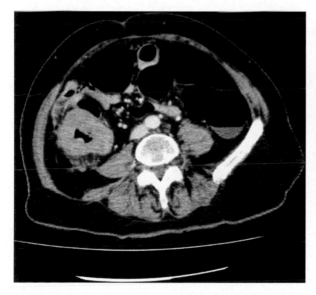

Image 1

R. Joarder et al., *Case Studies in Abdominal and Pelvic Imaging*, DOI: 10.1007/978-0-85729-366-4_24, © Springer-Verlag London Limited 2011

Answers

1. There is a large region of some tissue density in the caecal region (*arrow* Image 3). This maintains its position and morphology between the supine and prone sequences. There is no evidence of localised lymph node enlargement.
2. The findings are of a large tumour at this site, which given its size is most likely to be malignant.
3. CT imaging of the chest is required to complete staging. Direct visualisation and biopsy confirmation of malignancy may be required.

CT colography (virtual colonoscopy) has become an alternative method of investigation for patients who decline colonoscopy. One advantage of the technique over traditional barium enema as an investigation of the large bowel is the ability to review structures outside the bowel. It is possible to identify local or distant lymph node enlargement or distant metastatic disease, e.g. in the liver. If the examination is performed to investigate possible malignancy (as opposed to use for screening), intravenous contrast can be given and the chest included in one of the sequences, eliminating the need for the patient to return for completion staging.

A confident diagnosis of malignancy on virtual colonoscopy may be enough to proceed to operation. Patient factors may however necessitate a histological diagnosis before treatment is commenced.

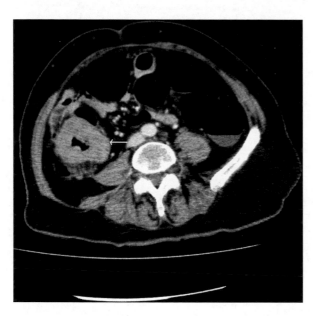

Image 3

Key Points

› CT colography is useful in patients unwilling to have traditional colonoscopy.
› Tumour staging can be performed in one examination.
› There is not always a need for histological confirmation.

A 20-year-old woman with suspected gallstones underwent US. This revealed a subtle iso-echoic mass distorting the adjacent intra-hepatic vessels in the right lobe of the liver. An MRI enhanced with Gadolinium-BOPTA was performed (Image 1, T1; Image 2, T2; Image 3, arterial phase; Image 4, portal venous phase; Image 5, equilibrium phase; and Image 6, hepatobiliary phase).

Questions

1. Describe the signal intensity of the lesion on T1 and T2.
2. Describe the enhancement pattern of the majority of the lesion.
3. Describe the enhancement pattern of the small central area of the lesion.
4. What is the diagnosis?

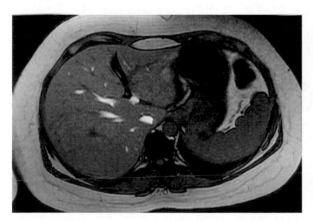

Image 1

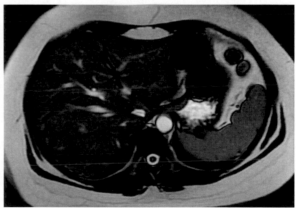

Image 2

R. Joarder et al., *Case Studies in Abdominal and Pelvic Imaging*,
DOI: 10.1007/978-0-85729-366-4_25, © Springer-Verlag London Limited 2011

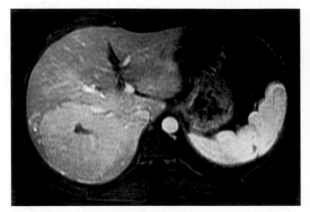

Image 3

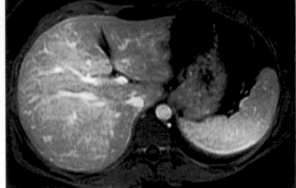

Image 5

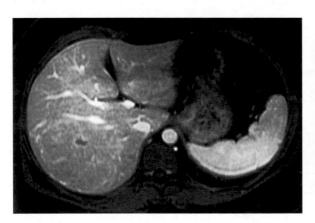

Image 4

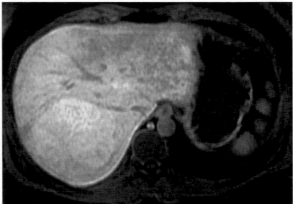

Image 6

Answers

1. Isointense compared to hepatic parenchyma on T1 and T2 apart from the small central area which is hypointense on T1 (*arrow* Image 7) and hyperintense on T2 (*arrow* Image 8).
2. There is marked enhancement in the arterial and portal venous phases, with washout in the equilibrium phase and moderate enhancement in the hepatobiliary phase (*star* Images 9–12).
3. Reduced enhancement in the arterial and portal phases, moderate enhancement in the equilibrium phase ('delayed enhancement') and iso-intense in the hepatobiliary phase (*arrow* Images 9–12).
4. Focal nodular hyperplasia (FNH).

This case shows the typical MRI signal characteristics and enhancement pattern of FNH. The main part of the mass is iso-intense on T1 and T2 and shows marked early enhancement which rapidly washes out followed by increased enhancement in the hepatobiliary phase (due to functioning hepatocytes in the mass – compare with Case 46). The small central area is the fibrous scar which is hypointense on T1 and hyperintense on T2 with delayed enhancement.

FNH is the second most common benign liver tumour (after haemangioma). It is thought to represent the non-neoplastic hyperplastic reaction of hepatocytes to a congenital vascular malformation. FNH derives its blood supply from the hepatic artery (accounting for its early enhancement and washout during dynamic

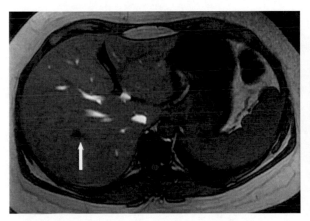

Image 7

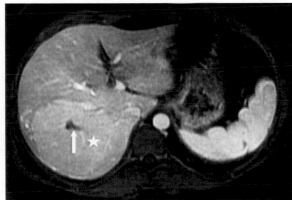

Image 9

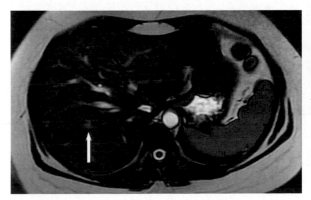

Image 8

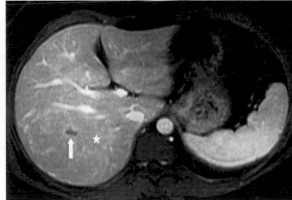

Image 10

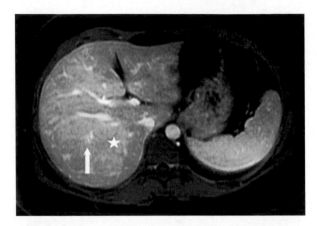

Image 11

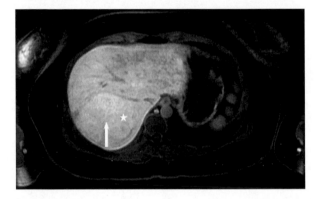

Image 12

enhancement). It contains functioning hepatocytes with impaired biliary drainage (accounting for its hepato-biliary phase enhancement – compare with Case 46).

Twenty percent of FNH, particularly larger lesions, have a central scar, which show delayed enhancement as described above.

Most FNH are small, well-circumscribed masses in the right lobe. Ninety percent are less than 5 cm, which makes the above case unusual.

Most FNH occur in young women of reproductive age – the oral contraceptive pill may promote their development but does not seem to stimulate growth (unlike hepatic adenomas which often grow during pregnancy or whilst taking the oral contraceptive pill).

Also, in distinction to hepatic adenomata, they do not necrose, bleed or undergo malignant change.

Most FNH can be confidently diagnosed on imaging (particularly gadolinium-BOPTA enhanced MRI or contrast-enhanced ultrasound). In a minority of patients, biopsy is performed but its interpretation can be difficult and may not be definitive.

Key Points

> FNH is a non-neoplastic reaction to a congenital vascular anomaly.
> FNH is a common benign tumour of women of reproductive age.
> No malignant potential or risk of haemorrhage or necrosis.
> CE MRI or CEUS is usually diagnostic.

Further Reading

Jang HJ, Yu H, Kim TK (2009) Imaging of focal liver lesions. Semin Roentgenol 44:266-282

A 74-year-old male presented with a 2-week history of left loin pain and macroscopic haematuria. An MDCT was performed (Images 1a–c and 2a and b).

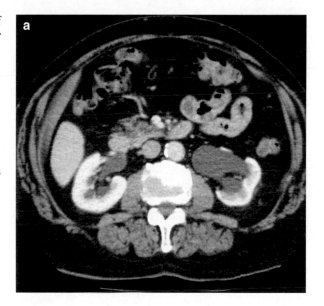

Image 1

Questions

1. What type of CT has been performed?
2. What does Image 1a show, what are the arrows pointing to in Images 1b and c?
3. When were the images acquired in Images 1a–c?
4. What do Images 2a and b show?
5. When were the images in 2a and b acquired?
6. What is the likely diagnosis?

R. Joarder et al., *Case Studies in Abdominal and Pelvic Imaging*,
DOI: 10.1007/978-0-85729-366-4_26, © Springer-Verlag London Limited 2011

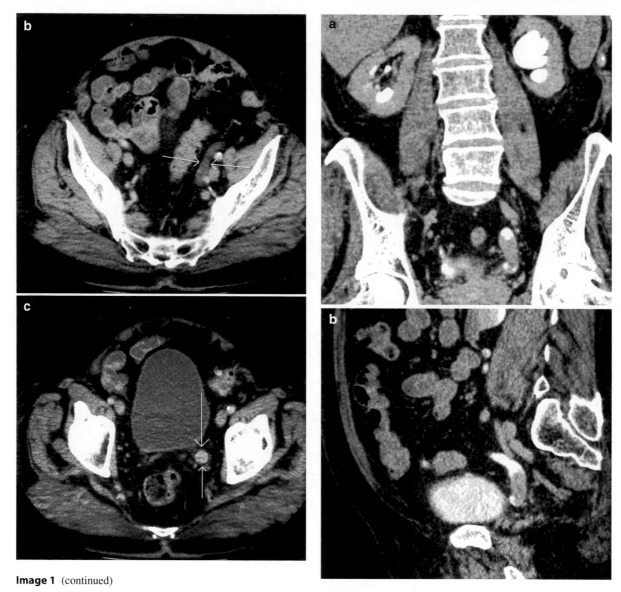

Image 1 (continued)

Image 2

Answers

1. A CT urogram (CTU).
2. A hydronephrotic left kidney.
   A dilated urine filled distal left ureter.
   The arrows are pointing to a solid soft tissue mass filling the more distal left ureter just above the left vesico-ureteric junction (VUJ).
3. During the arterial phase of intravenous contrast.
4. Coronal and sagittal reconstructions with a filling defect within the distal left ureter (Images 3a and b).

5. After a delay following IV contrast (approximately 15 m).
6. Transitional cell carcinoma (TCC) of the distal left ureter causing obstruction.

With the increasing access to MDCT more hospitals are performing CT urography (CTU) in place of the traditional intra-venous urogram (IVU) for both renal colic and persistent haematuria. Protocols for CT urography vary; however, in our institution we perform a two-phase study for haematuria acquiring scans during arterial and delayed (15 min post-contrast) phases of intravenous contrast [1]. During the arterial phase we can assess the renal parenchyma for neoplasms, which often enhance during this phase and also provide detail of the arterial supply to the affected kidney often required by the surgeon. The arterial phase also shows the renal collecting system unopacified to assess for calculi. We use the delayed phase to detect filling defects as in this case in the presence of TCC. We do not perform an unenhanced study unless we are only performing the scan for renal colic in which case it is the only scan we perform.

CTU also has the advantage of allowing the examination of the rest of the abdomen and pelvis. Albeit an arterial study, if a renal cell carcinoma is found metastases are often hypervascular and should be revealed. We would go back and scan the chest if a renal tumour is discovered.

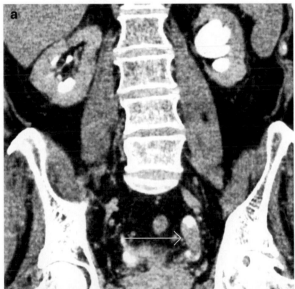

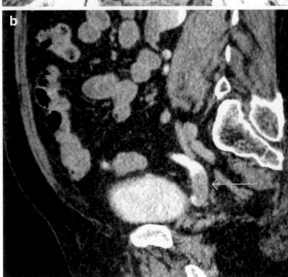

Image 3

Key Points

> CTU has replaced the more traditional IVU in many hospitals.
> CTU gives added information, e.g. more accurate assessment of a renal mass, detection of liver and lymph node metastases.
> Using a two-phase technique can help to keep radiation dose down.

Reference

1. Caoili E.M, Cohen R (2006) CT urography: technique and applications RSNA Categorical Course in Diagnostic Radiology: Genitourinary Radiology 11-22

An 82-year-old male was seen at the Emergency Department complaining of lethargy, shortness of breath and inability to pass urine.

He had a history of radiotherapy to his neck 6 months previously.

He was anaemic with an Hb of 7.6 and a raised white count. Urine culture shows *Proteus* species.

He underwent MDCT to exclude thromboembolic disease with venous phase imaging of the abdomen and pelvis.

Questions

1. What abnormalities do the three sections show?
2. What is the underlying diagnosis?

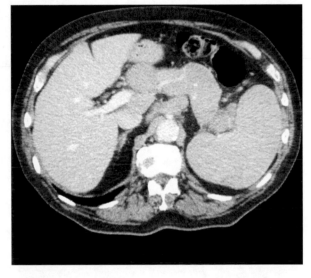

Image 2

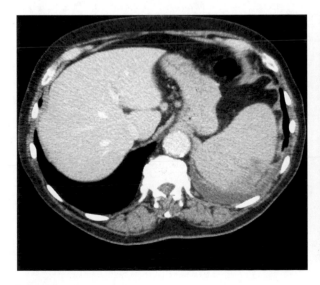

Image 1

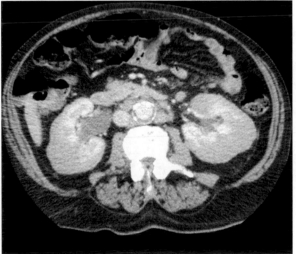

Image 3

R. Joarder et al., *Case Studies in Abdominal and Pelvic Imaging*,
DOI: 10.1007/978-0-85729-366-4_27, © Springer-Verlag London Limited 2011

Answers

1. There is a left-sided basal pleural effusion (Image 4 *long arrow*), and low attenuation abnormality peripherally in the spleen (*short arrow*). There is diffuse enlargement of the pancreas and lymph node enlargement at the porta hepatis (Image 5 *white arrow* and *black arrow*). There is diffuse enlargement of both kidneys with relatively poor peripheral enhancement (Image 6 *arrows*). There is also some prominence of the right renal pelvis.
2. The underlying diagnosis is lymphoma. The patient has had previous treatment for mantle cell lymphoma. This was nodal disease in the neck.

Some 40% of patients with lymphoma will have extra nodal disease, and it is more common in non-Hodgkin's lymphoma (NHL) than Hodgkin's lymphoma. Within the abdomen extra-nodal disease is most common in the spleen, and in order of decreasing frequency liver, GI tract, pancreas, abdominal wall, GU tract, adrenals, peritoneal cavity and biliary system.

Extra-nodal disease is said to be more common in mantle cell, lymphoblastic, Burkitt's and mucosa-associated lymphoid tissue (MALT) lymphomas. AIDS related and post-transplantation lymphoproliferative disorder (PTLD) are also more likely to be extra-nodal.

Pancreatic involvement usually occurs as a result of spread from nodes and is quoted as occurring in 30% of NHL. Renal involvement is less common (3–8%) but is the most common site of GU tract involvement. Lesions may be multiple or single discrete masses, direct spread or diffuse infiltration.

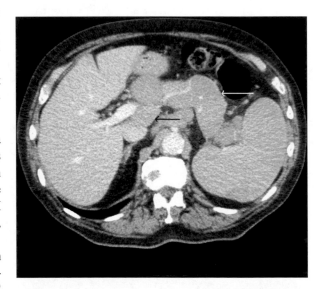

Image 5

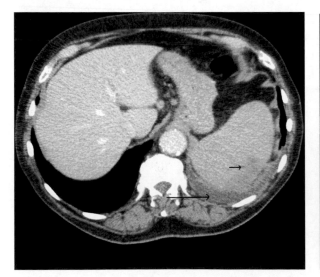

Image 4

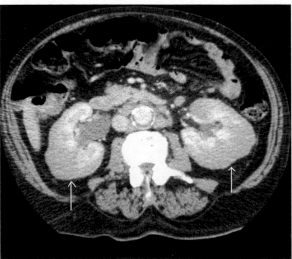

Image 6

Key Points

> Extra-nodal disease is common in lymphoma with the spleen as the commonest abdominal site.
> Diffuse organ enlargement is a feature of extra-nodal disease.

Further Reading

W. Lee, E. Lau, V. Duddalwar, A. Stanley, Y. Ho. Abdominal Manifestations of Extranodal Lymphoma: Spectrum of Imaging Findings. *AJR* 2008; 191:198–206

A 75-year-old male presented with right upper quadrant pain. US demonstrated gallstones in the gallbladder and elective laparoscopic cholecystectomy was performed. It was a difficult procedure and 2 days post-op a MDCT was performed for RUQ pain (Image 1). Bile was aspirated from the perihepatic collection and ERCP and biliary stenting was subsequently performed (Image 2). One year later the patient became jaundiced and an ERCP was performed (Image 3). Two years later the patient re-presented with recurrent fevers and intermittent abdominal pain. MDCT (Images 4 and 5) and MRI were performed (Image 6 T2 axial).

Questions

1. Describe the gallbladder fossa immediately after surgery (Image 1)
2. Describe the ERCP findings on Images 2 and 3
3. Describe and explain the findings on the MDCT and MRI (Images 4–6).

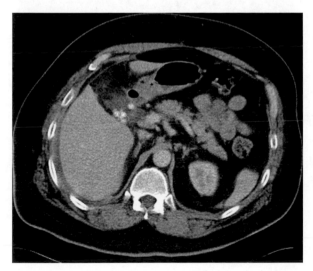

Image 1

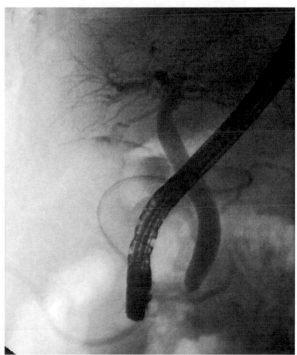

Image 2

R. Joarder et al., *Case Studies in Abdominal and Pelvic Imaging*, DOI: 10.1007/978-0-85729-366-4_28, © Springer-Verlag London Limited 2011

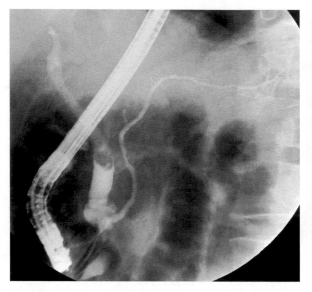

Image 3

Image 5

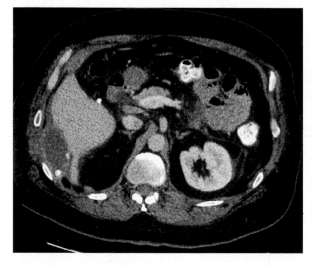

Image 4

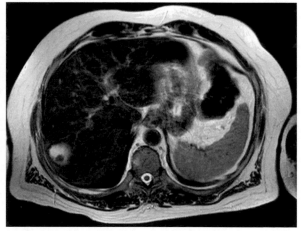

Image 6

Answers

1. There are gallstones in the gallbladder fossa – which have been 'dropped' during laparoscopic cholecystectomy (*arrows* Image 7)
2. The first ERCP shows contrast leaking from the biliary tree into the gallbladder fossa (*long arrow* Image 8) and down the surgical drain (*short arrows* Image 8). The second ERCP shows a gallstone in the common bile duct (*arrow* Image 9) which was removed.
3. The gallstones (*long arrows* Images 10–12) have moved from the gallbladder fossa and are now dispersed around the abdomen and surrounded by encapsulated fluid (*short arrows* Images 10–12).

This case demonstrates some of the complications of cholecystectomy.

First, the patient developed a bile leak. These are usually from the cystic duct remnant or small ducts of Luschka passing from the right lobe directly to the

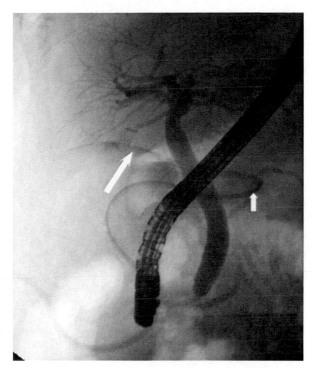

Image 8

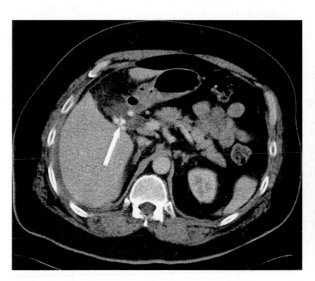

Image 7

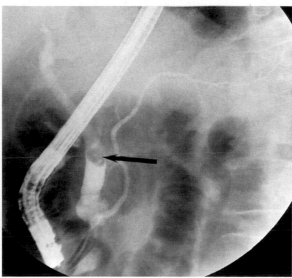

Image 9

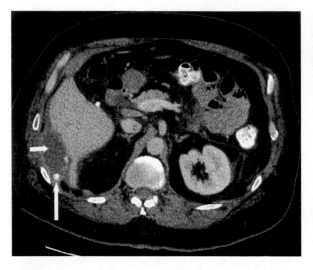

Image 10

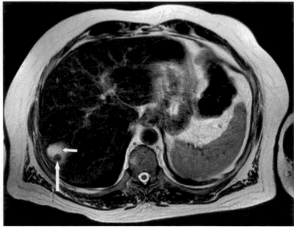

Image 12

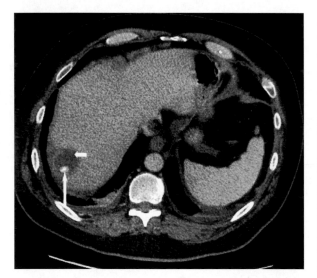

Image 11

gallbladder. As in this case, bile leaks usually respond to biliary stent insertion and fluid aspiration/drainage (particularly if the fluid is infected).

Second, the patient developed jaundice due to bile duct stones – this may have been missed during the work up before cholecystectomy, accidentally spilled into bile duct during the operation or formed in the CBD subsequent to the operation. The stone was removed endoscopically.

Third, the patient developed multiple intra-abdominal abscesses around 'dropped gallstones' that were spilled into the abdominal cavity during cholecystectomy. These were all removed and the abscesses drained surgically.

Key Points

> Cholecystectomy has occasional complications.
> Bile leaks usually respond to endoscopic biliary stent insertion.
> Jaundice after cholecystectomy is best investigated with MRCP as US has low sensitivity for bile duct stones.
> Dropped gallstones may be asymptomatic but can lead to abscess formation or other complications.

Further Readings

Pinkas H, Brady PG. (2008) Biliary leaks after laparoscopic cholecystectomy: time to stent or time to drain. Hepatobiliary Pancreat Dis Int 7(6):628-32

Singh AK, Levenson RB, Gervais DA, et al. (2007) Dropped gallstones and surgical clips after cholecystectomy: CT assessment. J Comput Assist Tomogr 31(5):758-62

A 76-year-old female presented to the Emergency Department with a 1-week history of not opening her bowels and abdominal pain. She had a background of chronic constipation. On examination she had a distended abdomen and a diffuse palpable mass. An AXR (Image 1) and CT of the abdomen (Images 2a–c) were performed.

Questions

1. What does the plain film in Image 1 show?
2. What is the sign demonstrated here?
3. What is the most likely diagnosis?
4. What can the CT add/exclude?

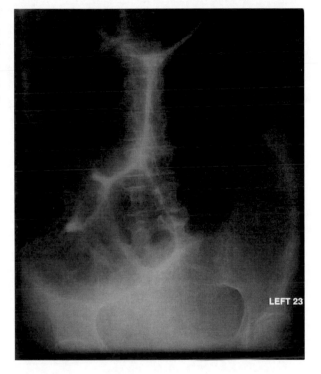

Image 1

R. Joarder et al., *Case Studies in Abdominal and Pelvic Imaging*, DOI: 10.1007/978-0-85729-366-4_29, © Springer-Verlag London Limited 2011

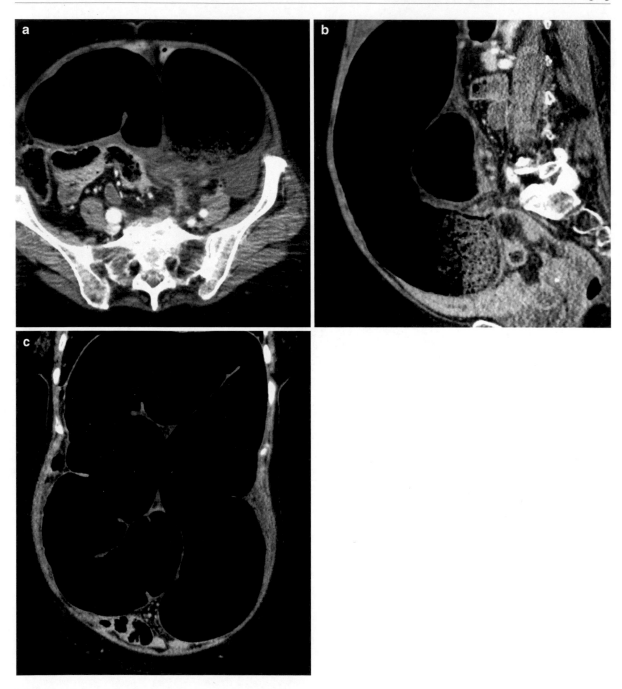

Image 2

Answers

1. Grossly distended sigmoid colon filling abdomen.
2. The 'coffee bean' sign [1] (Image 3, the *arrow* points to the central cleft of the coffee bean). This refers to the central opaque line caused by opposing distended loops of sigmoid up against the mesentery on a supine film.
3. Sigmoid volvulus.
4. The plain film is diagnostic in this case; however, if there is doubt a CT scan is a relatively non-invasive way of confirming the diagnosis, assessing for ischaemia and/or perforation and to look for other causes of pain and distension.

The *arrows* in Images 4a and b are pointing to the location of the twist seen as a 'bird's beak' shape. Image 4c demonstrates the CT equivalent of 'the coffee bean sign'.

Sigmoid volvulus is a common cause of large bowel obstruction. In the Western world it is the third leading cause after carcinoma and diverticular stricture and is particularly common in the elderly where there is often a background of chronic constipation and laxative use. In South America it is linked with Chagas disease and in Africa with a high fibre diet, the age group is often younger in these countries than in the West.

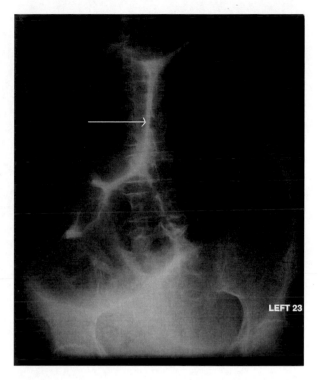

Image 3

There is a high mortality of around 20% particularly in the elderly patients seen in the West. Around 80% can be diagnosed on a supine AXR alone and therefore treated quickly with no need for further imaging.

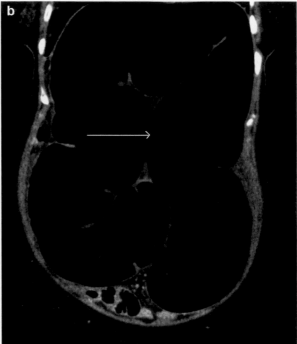

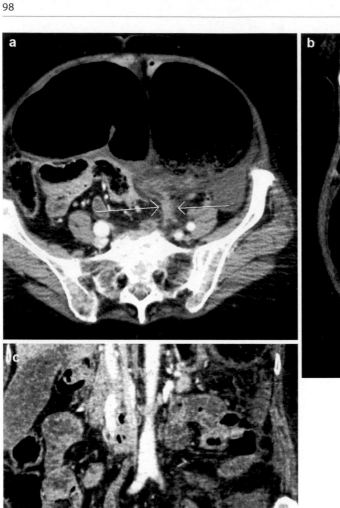

Image 4

> Eighty percent sigmoid volvulus can be diagnosed on a supine AXR.
> Look for the 'coffee bean' sign (Image 3)
> There is a 20% mortality and delay of treatment increases the risk of ischaemia and/or perforation.

Reference

1. Deborah Feldman (2000) The coffee bean sign. Radiology 216, 178-179

An 80-year-old presented to the Emergency Department with a history of acute onset headache. He also complained of chest pain that passed into his abdomen. He had a background history of emphysema and took warfarin for stable atrial fibrillation.

On examination he was hypotensive, without evidence of anaemia.

A chest X-ray was performed and then in view of the persisting hypotension a CT is requested.

Questions

1. What does the chest X-ray show?
2. What does the CT show?
3. What are the treatment options?

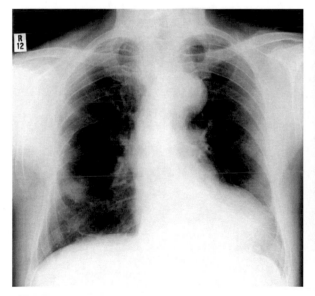

Image 1

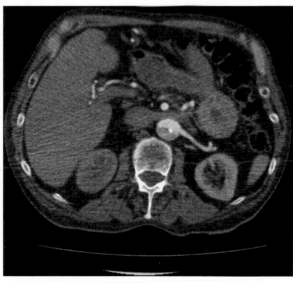

Image 2

R. Joarder et al., *Case Studies in Abdominal and Pelvic Imaging*, DOI: 10.1007/978-0-85729-366-4_30, © Springer-Verlag London Limited 2011

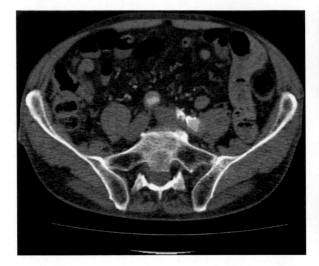

Image 3

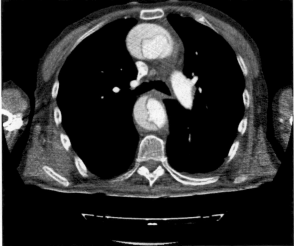

Image 4

Answers

1. The chest X-ray shows a degree of unfolding of the thoracic aorta with some widening of the region of the aortic root. There is also some rather ill-defined increased density in the right hemithorax projecting over the ninth posterior rib on the right.
2. Image 5 is at the level of the left renal artery. There is dissection of a normal calibre abdominal aorta (*black arrow*). Contrast is seen in the renal artery (*white arrow*). Image 3 is just below the level of the aortic bifurcation. The dissection continues into the common iliac vessels bilaterally.

   Image 6 through the thorax shows that the dissection involves both ascending and descending thoracic aorta. The ill-defined opacity seen on chest X-ray was also seen at another level and had the appearance of a coincidental lung neoplasm.
3. Given the extent of the dissection, medical management is the only option. A fenestration is an option if there is a significant ischaemia, for example in the

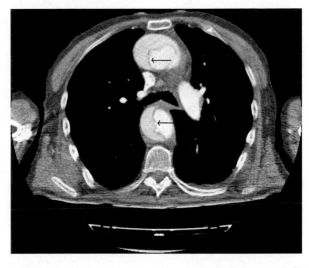

Image 6

intestines, leg or kidneys but does not help brain perfusion. Some centres attempt hybrid procedures where there is surgical repair/replacement of ascending and stent grafting distal to arch.

There is a dissection of the entire aorta passing into the iliac vessels. This is said to occur in 5% of thoracic aortic dissections. Termination is more commonly into the left iliac vessel with involvement of both quoted at around 10%. Prognosis, particularly in the absence of surgical intervention is very poor.

Diagnosis of abdominal aortic dissection extension in the acute setting is usually done by MDCT.

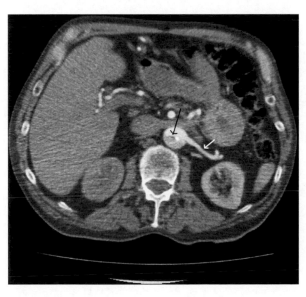

Image 5

Key Points

> Extension of a thoracic aortic dissection into the abdominal aorta occurs in a small number of cases.
> Prognosis is poor in the absence of a surgical treatment option.

A 50-year-old tee-total man presented with a short history of central abdominal pain. The abdomen was mildly tender but not peritonitic. The serum amylase was elevated. US showed no gallstones in the gallbladder and CT demonstrated pancreatic swelling, but no fluid collections or necrosis. A diagnosis of mild acute pancreatitis was made.

As the aetiology of the pancreatitis was unknown, MRCP was performed.

Questions

1. Describe the pancreatic ductal system
2. What is the diagnosis?

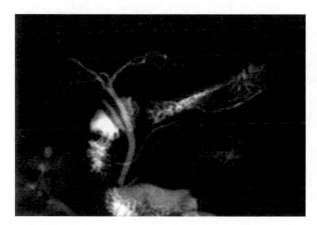

Image 1

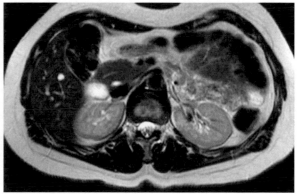

Image 2

R. Joarder et al., *Case Studies in Abdominal and Pelvic Imaging,*
DOI: 10.1007/978-0-85729-366-4_31, © Springer-Verlag London Limited 2011

Answers

1. The small ventral duct (*long arrow* Image 3) drains via the major papilla – this is also show in the ERCP images (Image 5). The main/dorsal pancreatic duct (*short arrows* image 3) drains via minor papilla lying proximally in the duodenum (*medium arrow* Image 3). The main pancreatic duct (*short arrow* Image 4) lies anterior to the common bile duct (*long arrow* Image 4) in the head of the pancreas.
2. Pancreas divisum.

Pancreas divisum is a congenital anomaly occurring in 5–10% of the population when the embryological ventral and dorsal parts of the pancreas fail to fuse. The embryological anatomy persists where the main pancreatic drainage (approximately 70%) is via the

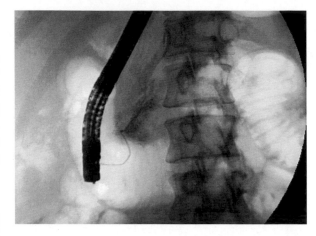

Image 5

dorsal duct through the accessory/minor papilla (lying cephalad/proximal to the major papilla in the duodenum) and the ventral duct drains via the major papilla.

The significance of pancreas divisum is uncertain and controversial. Some authors believe it predisposes to pancreatitis and obstructive pain [1] – possibly due obstruction of pancreatic juices as the minor/accessory duct is small or stenotic. Manometry has proved unreliable. Treatment with endoscopic sphincterotomy, or if unsuccessful, open surgery – including pancreatic duodenectomy has been proposed.

Other authors believe the pancreas divisum does not predispose to pancreatitis and the two occurring together is incidental [2].

Although ERCP is the 'gold standard' MRCP is commonly used to diagnose pancreas divisum. But again this is controversial, some authors demonstrating a low sensitivity [3] whilst others believe it to be accurate [4].

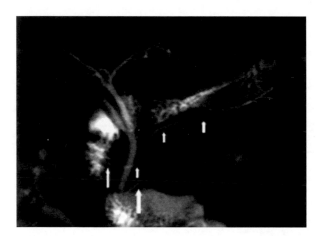

Image 3

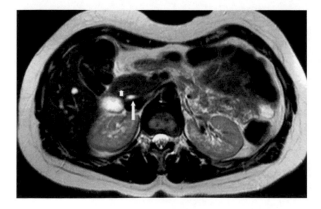

Image 4

Key Points

> Pancreas divisum occurs in 5–10% of the western population.
> The main pancreas drainage is via the dorsal duct and accessory papilla.
> Its relationship to pancreatits is controversial.
> It can be diagnosed by ERCP or MRCP (although sensitivity of MRCP may be suboptimal).

References

1. Cotton PB. (1980) Congential anomaly of pancreas divisum as cause of obstructive pain and pancreatitis. Gut 21:105-114
2. Delhaye M, Engleholm L, Cremer M. (1985) Pancreas divisum: congenital anatomical variant or anomaly? Contribution of endoscopic retrograde dorsal pancreatography. Gastroentorol 89 (5): 951-8
3. Carnes ML, Romagnuolo J, Cotton PB. (2008) Miss Rate of Pancreas Divisum by Magnetic Resonance Cholangio-pancreatography in Clinical Practice. Pancreas 37(2): 151-153
4. Bret PM, Reimhold C, Taourel P et al. (1996) Pancreas divisum: evaluation with MR cholangiopancreatography. Radiology 199:99-103

A 62-year-old male presented with obstructive jaundice and epigastric pain.

Questions

1. What type of examination has been performed?
2. What does it show?
3. What is the diagnosis?

R. Joarder et al., *Case Studies in Abdominal and Pelvic Imaging*,
DOI: 10.1007/978-0-85729-366-4_32, © Springer-Verlag London Limited 2011

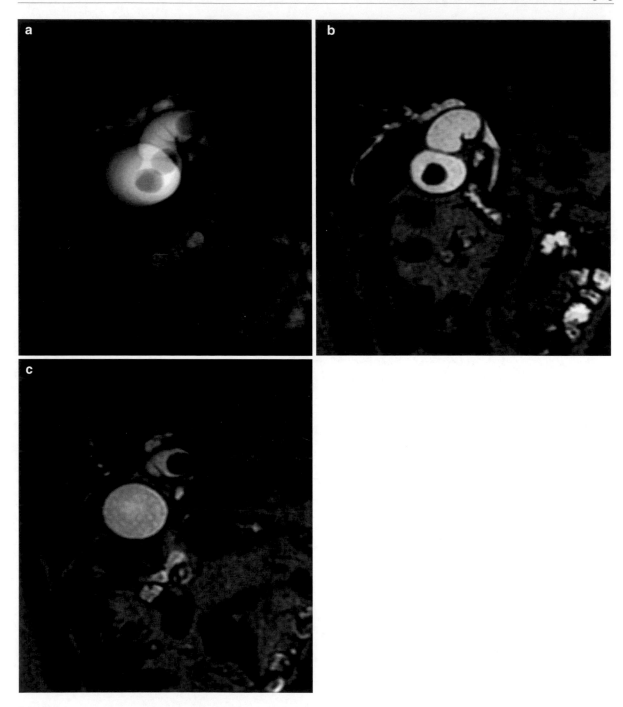

Image 1

Answers

1. A magnetic resonance cholangiopancreatogram (MRCP).
2. It shows dilated intrahepatic ducts (*long vertical arrows* Image 2), a normal calibre of common bile duct (*single, long horizontal arrow* Image 2), and gallstones with one gallstone within the neck of the gall bladder (*short oblique arrows* Image 2) responsible for obstruction of the common hepatic duct (CHD).
3. Mirizzi syndrome.

Mirizzi syndrome was first described in 1948 as obstructive jaundice caused by an impacted gallstone within either the cystic duct or the neck of the gallbladder (Hartmann's pouch) compressing the CHD [1]. It occurs in approximately 1% of patients with gallstones. Complications can include partial or complete erosion of the stone into the CHD resulting in a cholecystocholedochal fistula.

The original description classified these two scenarios of obstruction of the common hepatic duct alone as Type I and fistula formation as Type II.

A more recent classification was made in 1989 detailing the extent of fistula formation with respect to the circumference of the CHD: Type II 1/3, III 2/3 and IV complete destruction of the CHD [2].

The treatment is surgical; however, the exact type of operation will vary according to whether there is fistula formation or not. This level of detail may sometimes only be determined at surgery. However, it is important to diagnose Mirizzi syndrome from imaging where possible to assist surgical planning.

Key Points

> Recognition of Mirizzi syndrome is important to allow surgical planning and to avoid complications.
> Fistula formation may sometimes only be found at surgery.

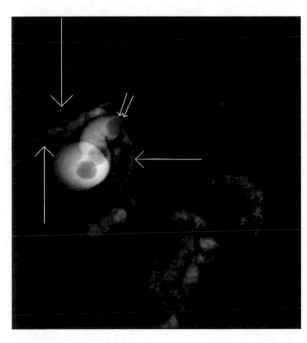

Image 2

References

1. Mirizzi PL (1948) Syndrome del conducto hepatico. J Int de Chir 1948, 8:731-3
2. Csendes A et al (1989) Mirizzi syndrome and cholecystobiliary fistula: A unique classification. Br J Surg 76: 1139-43

Further Reading

M. Safioleas et al (2008) Mirizzi Syndrome: an unexpected problem of cholelithiasis. Our experience with 27 cases. International Seminars in Surgical oncology 5:12

A 55-year-old attended the Emergency Department with a 3-week history of a swollen right leg. He also mentioned some episodes of fever and shivering and recent onset dysuria.

Examination showed a non-erythematous swollen leg. There was low-grade pyrexia, 37.9°C; ESR and CRP were mildly elevated. Urinalysis showed proteinuria only. Doppler US was negative for deep vein thrombosis.

He was started empirically on antibiotics for urinary sepsis whilst cultures were awaited. An out patient MDCT of his abdomen and pelvis was arranged.

Questions

1. What are the findings on the CT?
2. What do they represent?
3. What further investigations are required and what are the treatment options?

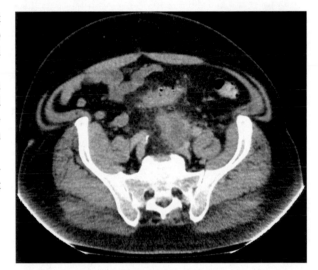

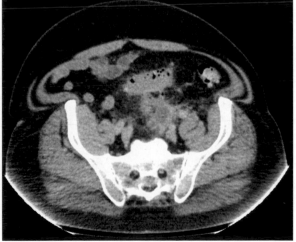

Image 2

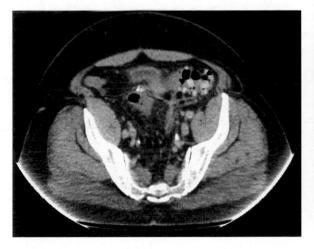

Image 1

Image 3

R. Joarder et al., *Case Studies in Abdominal and Pelvic Imaging*,
DOI: 10.1007/978-0-85729-366-4_33, © Springer-Verlag London Limited 2011

Answers

1. There is evidence of diverticular disease in the sigmoid region. There is ill-defined 6 × 5 cm mass consisting of alteration of attenuation adjacent to the bowel (Image 4 *black arrow*). This contains flecks of air (*white arrow*). There is extensive regional fatty stranding. The superior margin of the bladder is thickened and is closely related to the margin of the mass.
2. The findings represent an inflammatory mass in the left hemipelvis. This is likely to be related to the underlying diverticular disease. The proximity to and possible involvement of the bladder wall may explain the urinary symptoms.
3. Direct visualisation of the sigmoid region is required to exclude an underlying neoplastic process. Treatment is likely to be conservative in the first instance with antibiotics. Surgery for the underlying diverticular disease could be considered once the acute inflammation has resolved.

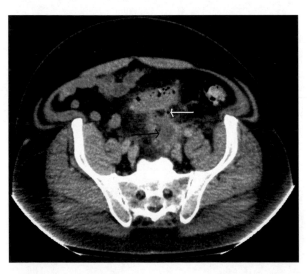

Image 4

Diverticular disease is a very common condition affecting the whole bowel. The colon and particularly the sigmoid region are most affected. In the USA, colonic diverticulosis is quoted as occurring in one-third of patients over 45 and up to two-thirds of those over 85. Risk factors seem to include a low fibre diet, inactivity and obesity.

Diverticulosis refers to the presence of diverticulae whilst diverticulitis represents a spectrum of inflammatory changes from subclinical localised inflammation to general peritonitis. With recurrent episodes, localised abscess formation may occur, which can involve adjacent organs. Fistula formation occurs: rates of 2.4–20% of cases are given. The majority of these are colovesical followed by colovaginal.

Elective surgical options include open and laparoscopic approaches. There remains debate as to the relationship between the number of episodes of uncomplicated diverticulitis and the timing of surgery.

Haemorrhage is a major complication and can be torrential. There is an increased incidence in patients on non-steroidal medications.

Key Points

> Diverticular disease is very common and may be unrecognised.
> Abscess formation occurs and may affect adjacent organs.
> Haemorrhage and fistula formation are important complications.

Further Reading

Sheth A, Longo W, Floch M, (2008) Diverticular disease and diverticulitis. Am J Gastroenterol 103(6): 1550-6

A 78-year-old male who had undergone anterior resection of a rectal carcinoma 3 days previously passed a large amount of fresh blood per rectum. This resulted in hypotension, tachycardia and required blood transfusion.

A CT angiogram (CTA) of the abdomen and pelvis was performed (Image 1, axial CT in arterial phase and Image 2, sagittal CT in arterial phase).

Questions

1. What abnormality does the CTA show?
2. What should be done next?

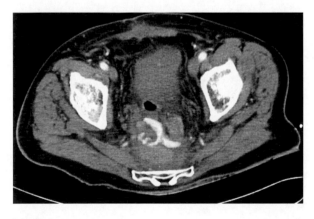

Image 1

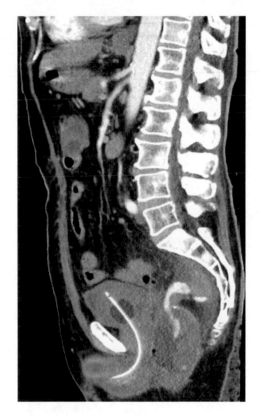

Image 2

R. Joarder et al., *Case Studies in Abdominal and Pelvic Imaging*,
DOI: 10.1007/978-0-85729-366-4_34, © Springer-Verlag London Limited 2011

Answers

1. Extravasation of contrast into the colon close to the surgical anastamosis (*arrows* Images 3 and 4).
2. Immediate transfer to the interventional radiology suite for transcatheter embolisation.

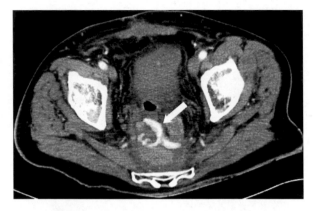

Image 3

Intra-arterial angiography demonstrated the bleeding from a branch of the anterior division of the internal iliac artery (*arrow* Image 5), which was selectively catheterized and embolised with gelatine sponge and metal coils (*arrow* Image 6).

GI bleeding that cannot be controlled endoscopically should be considered for transcatheter arterial embolisation (TAE). This is often preceded by CTA to demonstrate the site of bleeding and arterial anatomy – thus simplifying and speeding the embolisation. However, if no contrast extravasation is seen on the CTA then it is unlikely that the extravasation will be seen on angiography and embolisation of the bleeding vessel will not be possible. CTA is usually only performed when there are haemodynamic effects of blood loss, i.e. systolic BP less than 100 mmHg, tachycardia of greater than 100 bpm and blood transfusion of greater than 4 units in the preceding 24 h, as extravasation will usually only be identified during significant haemorrhage [1].

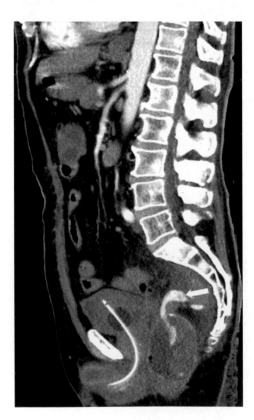

Image 4

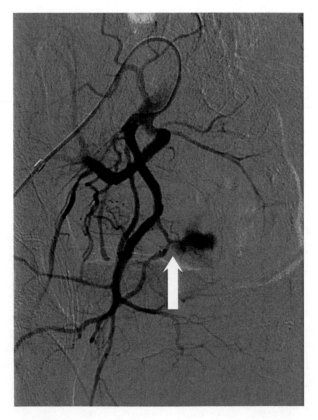

Image 5

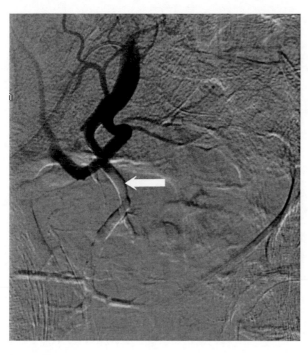

Image 6

> GI bleeding that is not controlled by endo-scopic means should be referred to IR.
> CTA is best performed when the patient is actively bleeding.
> If the CTA shows contrast extravasation, transcatheter embolisation should be attempted.

Reference

1. Anthony S, Milburn S, Uberoi R. (2007) Multi-detector CT: review of its use in acute GI haemorrhage. Clin Radiol 62(10): 938-49

A 66-year-old female who was initially investigated by the urologists for urinary incontinence (since settled) 3 years previously. These investigations included an US in year 1 (Image 1) and subsequent follow up with CT in years 2 and 3 (Images 2a–c and 3).

Questions

1. What does the first US in Image 1 show?
2. What do Images 2 and 3 show? Is there any significant difference?
3. What is the diagnosis?
4. What treatment has been performed?

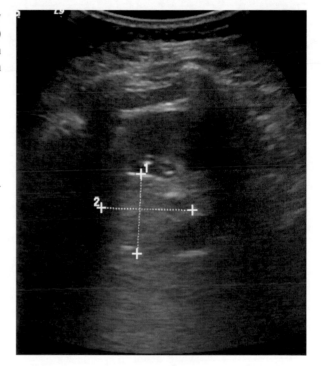

Image 1

R. Joarder et al., *Case Studies in Abdominal and Pelvic Imaging*,
DOI: 10.1007/978-0-85729-366-4_35, © Springer-Verlag London Limited 2011

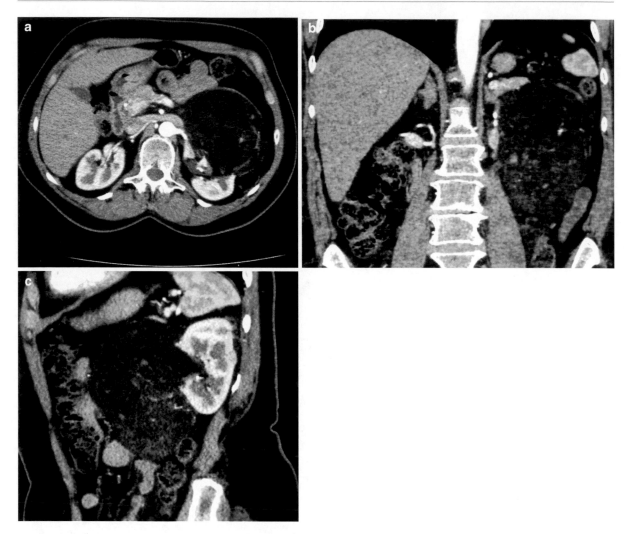

Image 2

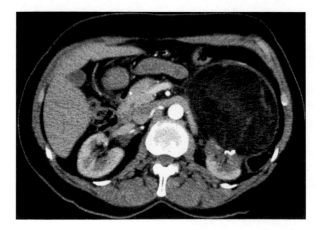

Image 3

Answers

1. US (year 1) showed a hyperechoic soft tissue mass arising from the anteriomedial aspect of the left kidney.
2. The first CT (year 2) shows a fatty soft tissue mass arising from the anterior aspect of the left kidney (Images 4a–c). The second CT, a year later, is found to be marginally bigger.
3. A renal angiomyolipoma.
4. Selective left renal artery embolisation of angiomyolipoma (Image 5) using particles and coils.

Renal angiomyolipomas are benign tumours but carry a risk of aneurysm formation and rupture. Angiomyolipomas tend to grow and when they do they become symptomatic. Also, as they grow the blood flow supplying it increases causing vessel dilatation and aneurysm formation. The main predictor for haemorrhage has been found to be tumour size [1]. Aneurysm size has also been found to be a predictor of rupture [2].

Arterial embolisation can be used, as in this case, for the treatment of symptomatic or enlarging angiomyolipomas to attempt to prevent further growth and spontaneous rupture. In this case, no aneurysm was identified and the angiomyolipoma had continued to enlarge.

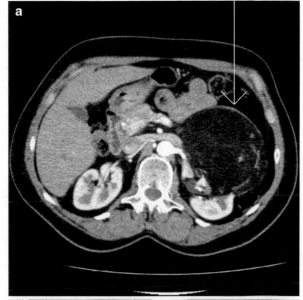
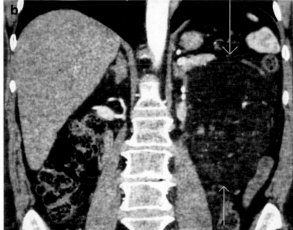
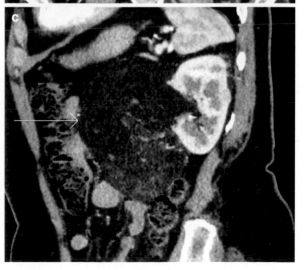

Image 4

Key Points

> Angiomyolipomas of the kidney are benign fatty tumours that can contain variable amounts of smooth muscle and blood vessels.

> Symptoms develop in 68–80%, if tumour size is >4 cm.

> Patients can present with acute pain associated with rupture due to haemorrhage.

> Treatment to prevent rupture should be considered in tumours greater than 4 cm.

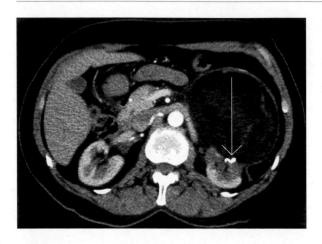

Image 5

References

1. Steiner MS et al (1993) The natural history of renal angio-myolipoma. J Urol 150:17782-1786
2. Yamakado K et al (2002) Renal Angiomyolipoma: Relation-ships between tumour size, aneurysm formation, and rupture. Radiology 225:78-82

An 80-year-old man was investigated in outpatients for right hypochondrial and epigastric pain. An OGD resulted in a positive CLO test and he was commenced on eradication therapy. An US of his upper abdomen was performed followed by an MDCT scan.

Questions

1. What does the ultrasound (Image 1) show?
2. What does the CT show?
3. What is the radiological diagnosis?
4. What are the treatment options?

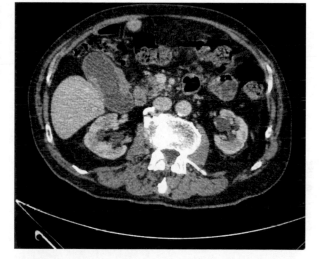

Image 2

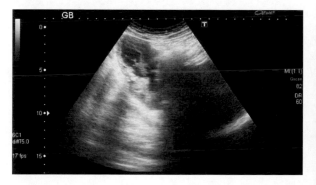

Image 1

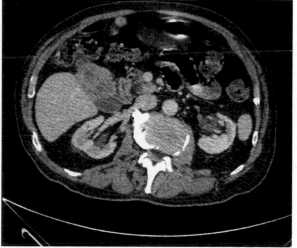

Image 3

R. Joarder et al., *Case Studies in Abdominal and Pelvic Imaging*, DOI: 10.1007/978-0-85729-366-4_36, © Springer-Verlag London Limited 2011

Answers

1. The ultrasound shows the gall bladder (GB) wall to be thickened and irregular (Image 4 *black arrow*). There are abnormal linear internal echoes within (*white arrow*). Other images show evidence of gall stones. The features may result from chronic inflammation, but a neoplastic process needs to be excluded.
2. The CT shows evidence of irregular thickening of the wall of the gall bladder. There is loss of definition of the margin of the gall bladder. There is also loss of definition of the plane of separation between gall bladder and liver with subtle alteration of attention within the liver adjacent to the GB fossa (Image 5 *black arrow*).
3. The radiological diagnosis is of gall bladder carcinoma. There is likely spread by direct invasion into the adjacent liver indicating T3 disease.

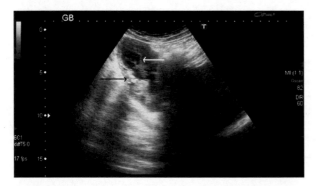

Image 4

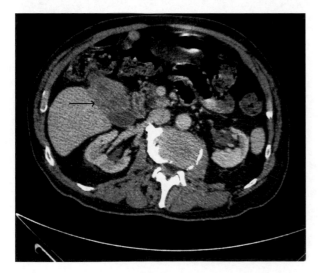

Image 5

4. Surgical resection is the only curative option. Recurrence is frequent particularly in advanced disease.

Gall bladder cancer is uncommon. Survival rates are low as disease is usually advanced by the time of presentation. Survival is best in patients where a carcinoma is found co-incidentally at cholecystectomy.

Associations include:

Porcelain gall bladder.
Inflammatory bowel disease (UC much more than Crohn's disease).
Gall stones – quoted rates for the presence of gall stones in patients with GB cancer are between 65% and 98%. However only 1% of individuals with gall stones develop cancer.

Radiological findings are of

- Focal or diffuse, but not generalised wall thickening;
- Polypoid mass of wide base;
- Mass replacing the whole GB.

Biliary distension is a frequent accompanying finding.

Surgical resection is the only curative option. The role of adjuvant chemo/radiotherapy is still controversial. Newer agents such as gemcitabine are felt by some to offer survival advantage as is adjuvant radiotherapy. Not all authors agree and the role of such treatment is currently unclear.

Key Points

> Gall bladder cancer is rare but has a poor prognosis as it usually presents late.
> Irregular focal wall thickening helps to differentiate cancer from more generalised thickening related to chronic inflammation.

Further Readings

Cho S, Kim S, Han S et al (2010) Adjuvant chemoradiation therapy in gallbladder cancer. J Surg Oncol 102(1):87-93
Kim W, Choi D, You D et al. (2010) Risk factors influencing recurrence, patterns of recurrence, and the efficacy of adjuvant therapy after radical resection for gallbladder carcinoma. J Gastrointest Surg.14(4):679-87

A 22-year-old male patient with long history of terminal ileal Crohn's disease underwent MDCT of the abdomen for right iliac fossa pain. Inflammatory markers and bowel habit were normal (Image 1, axial CT through right iliac fossa).

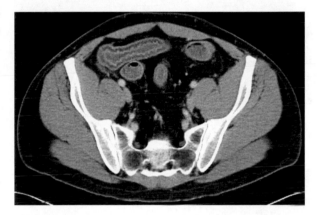

Image 1

Questions

1. Describe the appearance of the wall of the terminal ileum.
2. What is this sign?
3. What is its significance?

R. Joarder et al., *Case Studies in Abdominal and Pelvic Imaging*,
DOI: 10.1007/978-0-85729-366-4_37, © Springer-Verlag London Limited 2011

Answers

1. High attenuation of inner (*short arrow* Image 2) and outer layer (*long arrow*) of bowel wall with fat density (*medium arrow*) interposed between these two layers.
2. The 'fat halo sign'.
3. Chronic inflammatory bowel disease.

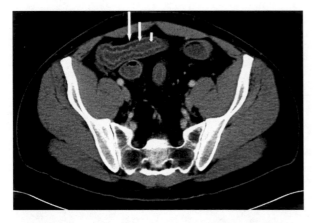

Image 2

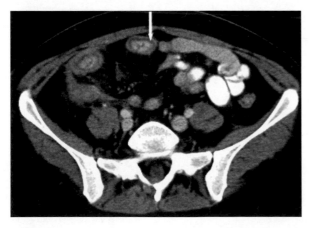

Image 3

The 'fat halo sign' describes the appearance of thick-walled large- or small-bowel wall with a layer of fat attenuation (less than 10 Hounsfield units [HU]) between the soft tissue attenuation inner and outer layers. The findings are due to fatty infiltration of the submucosa.

This sign is described most commonly in chronic inflammatory bowel disease – ulcerative colitis or Crohn's – but can also be seen in graft versus host and during cytoreductive therapy.

Intramural fat can be seen in up to 20% of patients with no gastro-intestinal disease, but in these 'normal' individuals the fatty layer is very thin.

The 'fat halo sign' should not be confused with the 'target sign' seen in acute bowel inflammation where there is also thickening of the bowel wall and low attenuation submucosa between higher attenuation inner and outer bowel wall. However in the 'target sign' the submucosa is oedematous and therefore of low attenuation, but not as low as fat and has a positive Hounsfield value (*arrow* Image 3 – active acute small bowel Crohn's disease).

Key Points

> 'Fat halo sign' is due to fatty infiltration of the submucosa of the bowel wall.
> It is seen in chronic inflammatory bowel disease.
> It is different from the 'target sign' of oedematous, low attenuation submucosa seen in active bowel inflammation.

Further Readings

Ahualli J. (2005) The Target Sign. Radiology 234:549-550
Ahualli J. (2007) The Fat Halo Sign. Radiology 242:945-946

An 80-year-old female presented with several years of headaches, tiredness and night sweats. She also complained of cramps in the hands and feet. She has been treated for hypertension by her GP for many years. An MDCT of the upper abdomen was performed (Images 1a and b).

Questions

1. What do Images 1a and b show?
2. What is the most likely diagnosis given the history?

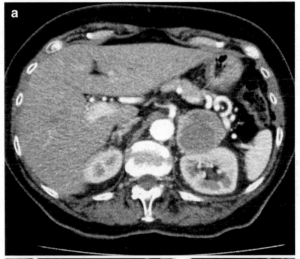

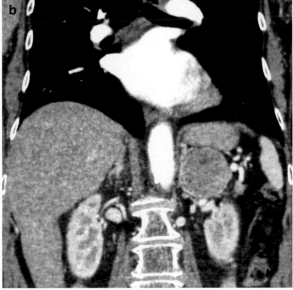

Image 1

R. Joarder et al., *Case Studies in Abdominal and Pelvic Imaging*,
DOI: 10.1007/978-0-85729-366-4_38, © Springer-Verlag London Limited 2011

Answers

1. A large mass expanding the left adrenal gland (*vertical arrow* Images 2a and b), separate from the left kidney. The right adrenal gland is normal in appearance (*horizontal arrows* Images 2a and b).
2. A pheochromocytoma.

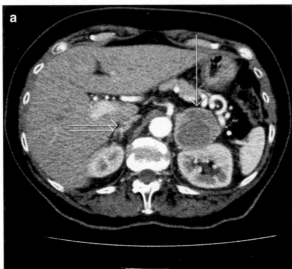

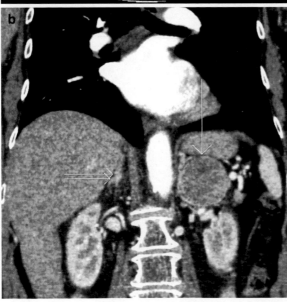

Image 2

Pheochromocytomas are rare catecholamine secreting tumours. Ten percent are asymptomatic, 10%, are benign and unilateral, 10% can be bilateral and malignant and 10% are hereditary. Classical clinical symptoms and signs are of hypertension, often episodic and difficult to treat with palpitations, headaches and hot flushes.

They are often diagnosed as an incidental finding on CTs performed for other reasons. They can cause a cardiovascular crisis if the diagnosis is not made therefore delaying treatment.

They are characteristically solid, hypervascular masses within the adrenal gland; however, can have many varied appearances. On CT they can be heterogeneous, solid or cystic complex masses and can show calcification. Most have attenuation higher than 10 HU (Houndsfield units), but can rarely contain enough fat to confuse them with the more common adrenal tumours – adenomas. Small tumours can be quite homogeneous. It is therefore important to consider the diagnosis in a patient with an adrenal mass and hypertension. Biochemical confirmation is mandatory.

Key Points

> 10 percent asymptomatic, 10% benign and unilateral, 10% bilateral and malignant, 10% hereditary.
> Often an incidental finding on CT.
> Usually solid and hypervascular but can be very variable in appearance.
> Can contain fat and be mistaken for an adenoma.
> Always consider if an adrenal mass is seen in a patient with a history of hypertension.

Further Reading

Michael Blake et al (2004) Pheochromocytoma: an imaging chameleon. Radiographics 24, S87-S99

Case 39

A 37-year-old female was assessed in the Emergency Department following a road traffic accident. She had an altered level of consciousness and bruising to her abdomen. Further evaluation was made by MDCT including her head and chest, abdomen and pelvis. The head CT showed no intracranial haemorrhage or evidence of fracture.

Questions

1. What does the CT abdomen show?
2. What are the complications of this procedure?
3. What is the long-term success rate?

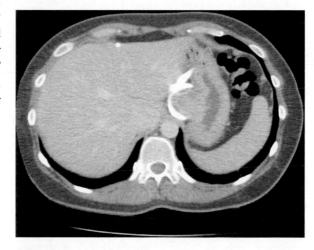

Image 2

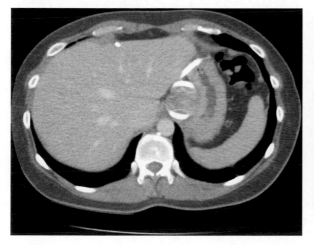

Image 1

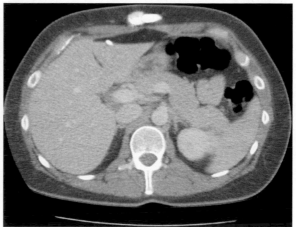

Image 3

R. Joarder et al., *Case Studies in Abdominal and Pelvic Imaging*,
DOI: 10.1007/978-0-85729-366-4_39, © Springer-Verlag London Limited 2011

127

Answers

1. The CT shows no evidence of traumatic injury. There is high attenuation material around the stomach with a curvilinear high attenuation passing to the anterior abdominal wall (Image 4). The findings represent laparoscopic adjustable gastric banding with an adjustment device in the anterior abdominal wall. The stomach is divided into two pouches using an adjustable silicone band. This creates a small area of approximately 15 mL. The band is connected to a port in the anterior abdominal wall allowing adjustment of the band (Image 5 *black arrow*).

2. Complications can be divided into short- and long-term.

   Short-term complications include gastric perforation, acute stomal stenosis and band slippage. Long-term complications include band erosion and chronic perforation, chronic stomal stenosis, and port and band complications such as catheter malfunction, or failure of port catheter or catheter band connection.

3. Long-term (5 years plus) success rates are quoted as mean excess weight loss in the range of 60%.

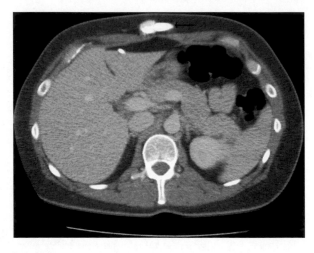

Image 5

Surgery aimed at weight loss/control (bariatric surgery) has two approaches – restriction and bypass. Restriction aims to reduce the volume of the stomach whereas bypass aims to generate reduced absorption by shortcutting part of the bowel. The procedures are those of laparoscopic adjustable gastric banding and laparoscopic Roux-en-y gastric bypass.

Long term success rates for the latter are quoted as being higher, although there are also higher rates of morbidity and mortality.

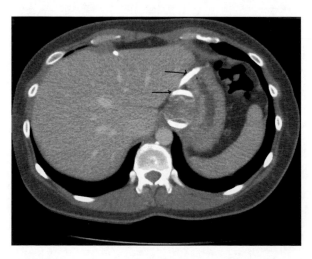

Image 4

> ## Key Points
>
> > Patient's previous surgical histories may be occult.
> > Bariatric surgery is becoming increasingly common.

Further Reading

Prosch H, Tscherney R, Kriwanek S, Tscholakoff D (2008) Radiographical imaging of the normal anatomy and complications after gastric banding. Br J Radiol. 81(969):753-7

A 40-year-old male presented with several days history of increasing dyspnoea. On examination the left side of the chest was hyper-resonant with no breath sounds. A pneumothorax was suspected and chest X-ray was performed. As insertion of an intercostal chest drain was being arranged by, the duty surgeon reviewed the chest X-ray and requested a MDCT of the chest and abdomen (Image 1, chest X-ray; Image 2, scanogram of CT; Image 3, coronal CT of chest (lung windows); Image 4, axial CT of upper abdomen and Image 5, coronal CT of upper abdomen).

Questions

1. Why did the surgical registrar stop the chest drain insertion?
2. What specific past history should be sought?
3. What is the diagnosis?

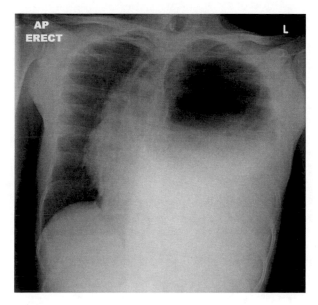

Image 1

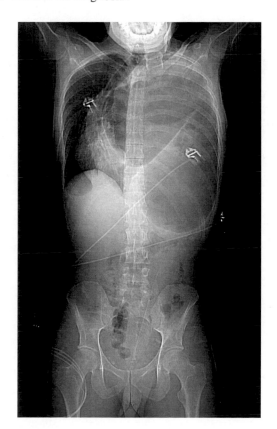

Image 2

R. Joarder et al., *Case Studies in Abdominal and Pelvic Imaging*, DOI: 10.1007/978-0-85729-366-4_40, © Springer-Verlag London Limited 2011

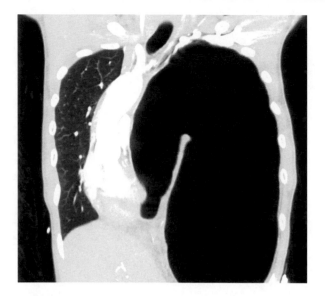

Image 3

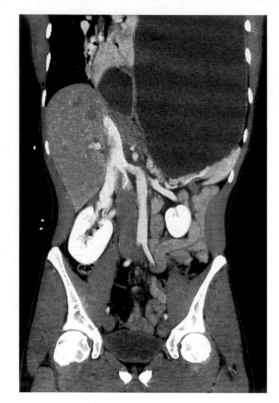

Image 5

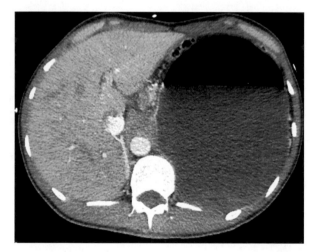

Image 4

Answers

1. The chest X-ray does not show a pneumothorax – although there are no left lung markings and the mediastinum is deviated to the right, no lung edge can be seen and the lower half of the hemi-thorax is of soft tissue or fluid density (*star* Image 6). The surgeon suspected an abnormality of the diaphragm such as eventration or rupture.
2. Any previous significant trauma – on direct questioning the patient reported a high-speed road traffic accident some months before.
3. Delayed diaphragmatic rupture. The CT shows herniation of the air and fluid filled stomach into the left hemi-thorax (*arrows* Images 7–10).

Diaphragmatic rupture can be from blunt or penetrating injury. Surgical repair is mandatory as there is a high chance of subsequent significant morbidity from herniation of abdominal contents into the chest. Occasionally, diaphragmatic rupture may go unrecognised and present sometime later. In this case, the diaphragmatic rupture was eventually recognised and

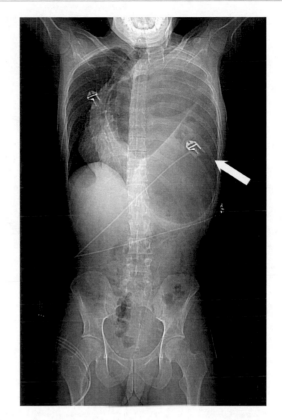

Image 7

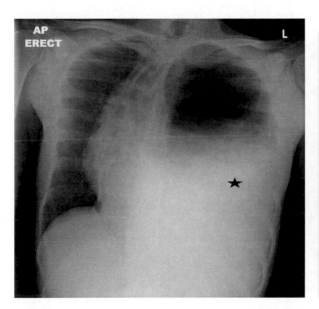

Image 6

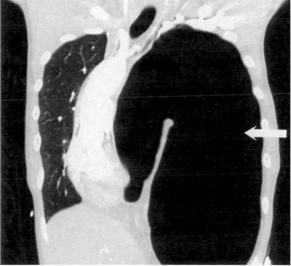

Image 8

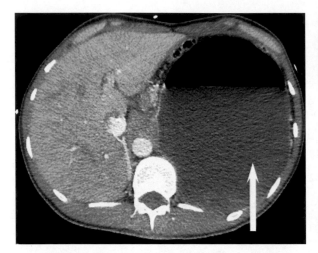

Image 9

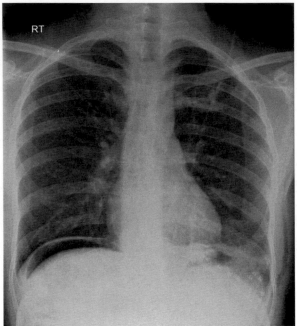

Image 11

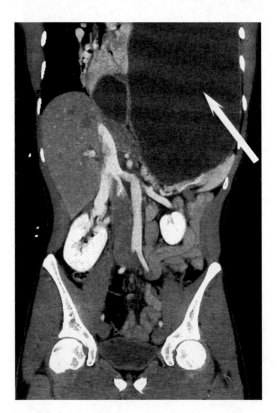

Image 10

repaired laparoscopically (Image 11 – CXR the day after surgery demonstrating re-expansion of the right lung and the abdominal contents below the diaphragm). There are several reports of chest drains being inserted into herniated stomachs which had been mistaken for a pneumothoraces).

The diagnosis of diaphragmatic rupture can be difficult on imaging. MDCT is the preferred modality– the multiplanar reconstructions of MDCT are particularly helpful – signs include diaphragmatic discontinuity, stomach herniation, 'dependent viscera' sign, 'abdominal organ herniation' sign, diaphragm thickening, or more than 4 cm elevation of one side of the diaphragm [1].

Key Points

> Although much less common, diaphragmatic rupture should be considered when a pneumothorax is seen on CXR.
> A history of trauma should be sought.
> Diaphragmatic rupture should be repaired surgically as there is a high incidence of significant morbidity.

Reference

1. Chen HW, Wong YC, Wang LJ, et al. (2010) Computed tomography in left sided and right sided blunt diaphragmatic rupture: experience with 43 patients. Clin Radiol 65(3); 206-12

Further Readings

Eren S, Kantarci M, Okur A. (2006) Imaging of diaphragmatic rupture after trauma. Clin Radiol 61:467-77

Rashid F, Chakrabarty MM, Singh R et al. (2009) A review on delayed presentation of diaphragmatic rupture. World J Emerg Surg 21;4:32

A 41-year-old male admitted on at least two occasions to Emergency Department with malaena and a significant drop in Hb. Upper GI endoscopy and colonoscopy were normal. On his third admission with further malaena a CT of the abdomen and pelvis (Images 1a and b) and an isotope-labelled red cell scan (Image 2) were performed.

Questions

1. What does the *arrow* in Image 1a and b show?
2. What does the posterior view of the red cell scan in Image 2 show?
3. What is the most likely diagnosis?

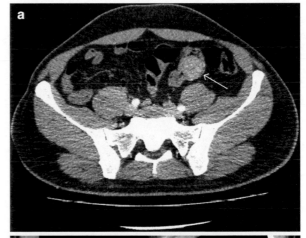

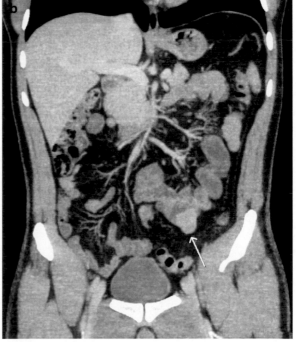

Image 1

R. Joarder et al., *Case Studies in Abdominal and Pelvic Imaging*,
DOI: 10.1007/978-0-85729-366-4_41, © Springer-Verlag London Limited 2011

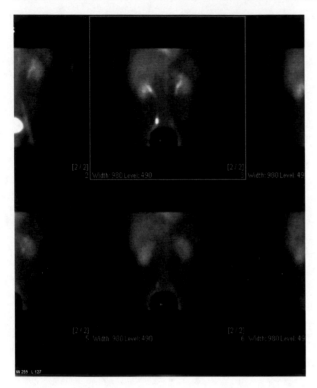

Image 2

Answers

1. A round, well-defined enhancing mass within the ileum.
2. There is increased activity within the left lower quadrant (Image 3).
3. A small bowel gastrointestinal stromal tumour (GIST).

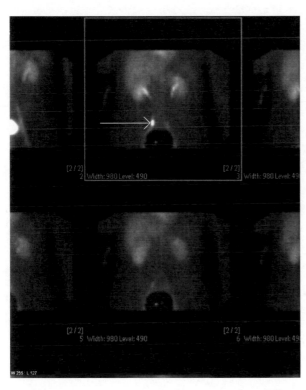

Image 3

GISTs are more common within the stomach, but do occur within the small bowel and can present with a GI bleed.

GISTs are a subset of GI mesenchymal tumours of varying differentiation and originate from the muscularis propria of the intestinal wall. The older medical literature referred to these as leiomyomas or leiomyosarcomas. They are usually found in the stomach, but can be found anywhere along the GI tract, the second most common site is the small bowel. Small- and low-grade tumours rarely metastasize; large- and high-grade tumours metastasize to the liver and peritoneum most commonly.

Radiologically, they are well-defined round lesions that appear to arise from the stomach or small bowel wall.

Key Point
› Think of a small bowel cause of GI bleeding, if OGD and colonoscopy are negative.

Case 42

An 80-year-old male was seen in medical outpatients. He gave a short history of a burning abdominal pain. There was no history of change of appetite or weight loss. Routine bloods showed a mild anaemia. An upper GI endoscopy and MDCT of the abdomen are arranged.

Questions

1. What does the CT show?
2. How is this disease staged?

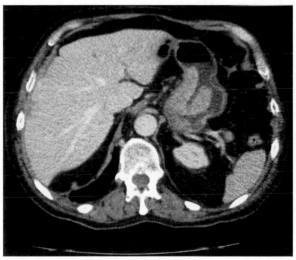

Image 1

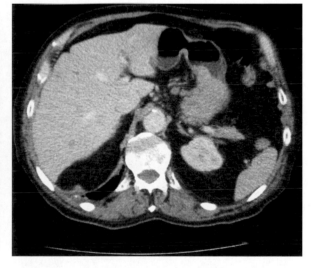

Image 2

R. Joarder et al., *Case Studies in Abdominal and Pelvic Imaging*,
DOI: 10.1007/978-0-85729-366-4_42, © Springer-Verlag London Limited 2011

Answers

1. The CT shows a soft tissue attenuation mass related to the proximal portion of the stomach (Image 3 *black arrow*). This is in keeping with a neoplastic process. It can sometimes be difficult to differentiate benign and malignant lesions within the stomach purely on CT appearance. Given the patient's age and the clinical history, a malignant process is most likely. Biopsy at endoscopy confirmed adenocarcinoma.

There are enlarged lymph nodes in the left gastric region (Image 4 *white arrow*), which would also favour a radiological diagnosis of malignancy.

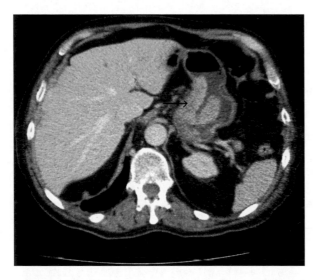

Image 3

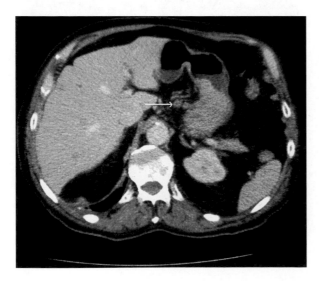

Image 4

2. Tumour staging for the primary disease is as follows:

   T1 tumour invades lamina propria or submucosa.

   T2 tumour invades muscularis propria or subserosa.

   T3 tumour penetrates serosa without invasion of adjacent structures.

   T4 tumour invades adjacent structures.

Lymph nodes staging is based upon number of positive nodes (rather than location).

   N1 1–6 regional nodes

   N2 7–15 nodes

   N3 greater than 15 nodes involved

Pre-operative staging of the tumour by CT is less reliable than by endoscopic ultrasound. Recent use of thinner sections and multiplanar reformat with newer CT technology had shown some improvement.

Positron emission tomography (PET) has the advantage of being a 'functional' form of imaging detecting uptake of molecules into cells. Most commonly this is fluorine 18–labelled deoxy-glucose (FDG). This seems to be most useful for determination of respectability. Currently, complete resection with the removal of local nodes is thought to be the only curative option for gastric cancer. PET, however, suffers from a lack of spatial resolution, which makes it less useful in local and nodal staging.

In vitro MRI studies have some promise in terms of local 'T' staging.

A combination of techniques may be required to optimise pre-operative staging.

Key Points

> The treatment pathway in stomach cancer depends upon the staging.

> CT staging of stomach cancer is more useful for lymph node disease than for T staging.

Further Reading

Lim J, Yun M, Kim M-J et al (2006) CT and PET in Stomach Cancer: Preoperative Staging and Monitoring of Response to Therapy. RadioGraphics 26:325-329

Case 43

A 78-year-old female with a history of previous anterior resection for Dukes A rectal cancer presented with several weeks of progressive nausea, vomiting and weight loss. OGD was normal apart from food debris in the oesophagus, stomach and duodenum. A barium follow-through was performed (Image 1). Subsequently, an MDCT of the abdomen and pelvis with oral contrast and IV contrast (portal venous phase) was performed (Image 2 *axial*).

Questions

1. What is the point of obstruction on the barium follow-through?
2. What is the differential diagnosis for this appearance?
3. What does the CT show?
4. What is the diagnosis?

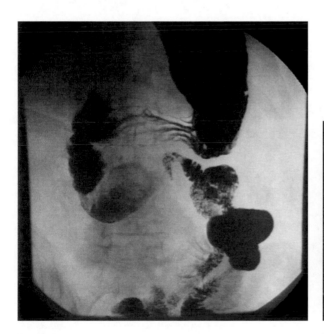

Image 1

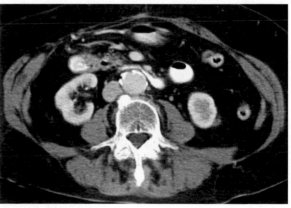

Image 2

Answers

1. The obstruction is at the junction of the third and fourth parts of the duodenum (*arrow* Image 3).
2. Intrinsic mass, i.e. duodenal carcinoma; extrinsic mass, i.e. pancreatic cancer; adjacent lymphadenopathy; or extrinsic compression by adjacent structure such as superior mesenteric artery (SMA).
3. The CT demonstrates compression of the third part of the duodenum as it passes through the small gap between the SMA and aorta (*arrow* Image 4).
4. SMA syndrome (also known as Wilkie's syndrome) which is compression and obstruction of the duodenum by the reduced angle between the SMA and aorta.

SMA or Wilkie's syndrome is a rare cause of vomiting and weight loss secondary to obstruction of the third part of the duodenum by the SMA. The syndrome is often precipitated by rapid weight loss (due to a variety

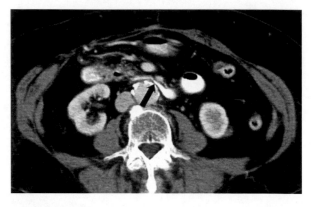

Image 4

of medical or psychiatric conditions), which reduces the angle between the SMA and aorta. The weight loss is then perpetuated by the duodenal obstruction which also causes nausea and vomiting. Diagnosis is often delayed, but should be considered when a young adult presents with weight loss and vomiting.

Treating the precipitating cause and surgery, in the form of open or laparoscopic doudenojejunostomy, may be necessary.

> **Key Points**
>
> › SMA syndrome is a rare cause of duodenal obstruction.
> › It should be considered in young adults presenting with weight loss, nausea and vomiting.

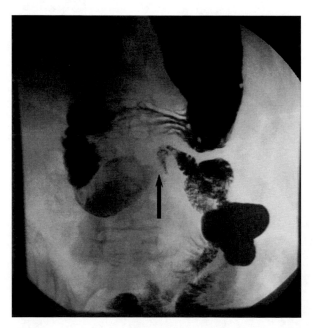

Image 3

Further Readings

Jain R. (2007) SMA syndrome. Curr treat options Gastroenterol 10(1):24-27
Merret ND et al 2009 Superior mesenteric syndrome: diagnosis and treatment strategies J Gastrointest Surg; 13(2):287-92

A 67-year-old male with a previous history of pancreatitis was under follow-up by the gastroenterologists. This follow-up involved serial CTs (Images 1a–c and 2a–c) a year apart.

Questions

1. What is the abnormality that is under review shown on the original CT on Images 1a–c?
2. How has this changed in appearance on the review CT scan 1 year later (Images 2a–c)?

R. Joarder et al., *Case Studies in Abdominal and Pelvic Imaging*,
DOI: 10.1007/978-0-85729-366-4_44, © Springer-Verlag London Limited 2011

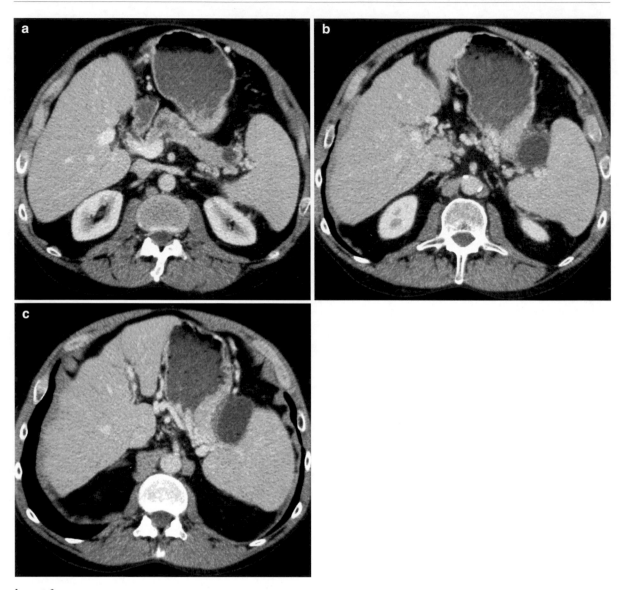

Image 1

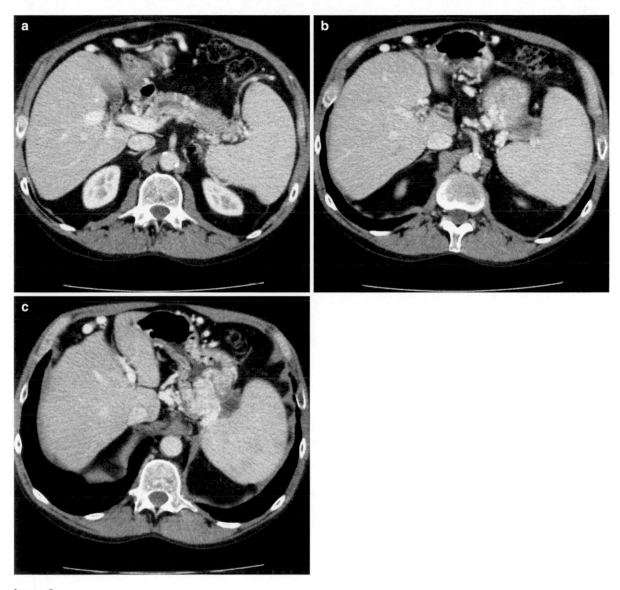

Image 2

Answers

1. There is a pancreatic pseudocyst within the tail of the pancreas (Image 3a).
2. There is now a fistula between the pseudocyst and the stomach in the region of the greater curve (Image 3b). The pseudocyst has now largely drained into the stomach. There is some associated thickening of the wall of the residual cyst in keeping with inflammatory change.

One treatment for troublesome painful pseudocysts is to actively create a fistula between the cyst and the stomach endoscopically. However, in this case the patient was relatively asymptomatic and had been followed up with imaging. The pseudocyst had spontaneously ruptured into the stomach with no associated symptoms. Spontaneous rupture into the stomach is rare and can be associated with significant bleeding, which may require surgery or embolisation. Uncomplicated rupture is even rarer, but has been described [1].

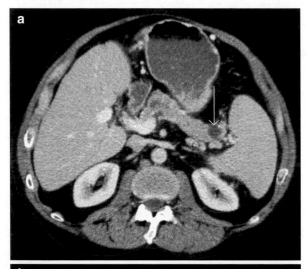

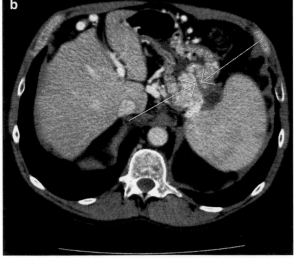

Image 3

Key Points

> The natural history of a pseudocyst includes resolution. Spontaneous rupture into the stomach is well reported, but rare.
> Spontaneous rupture is usually associated with life threatening bleeding.
> Uncomplicated rupture is even more unusual.

Reference

1. M F Mir et al (2009) Uncomplicated spontaneous rupture of the pancreatic pseudocyst into the Gut-CT documentation: A series of two cases; Gastroenterol 15:135-6

An 87-year-old woman was admitted to hospital following a fall. Her falls were longstanding with a recent increase in frequency.

She was seen in outpatients 6 months previously for investigation of anaemia, and declined colonoscopy.

As an inpatient she gave a recent history of increasing upper abdominal discomfort. She was noted to be pyrexial.

An US of the upper abdomen is followed by MDCT of the abdomen and pelvis.

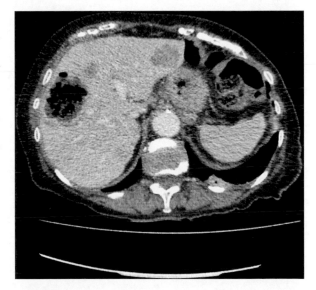

Image 2

Questions

1. What does the ultrasound show (Image 1)?
2. What does the CT show?
3. What is the most likely diagnosis?

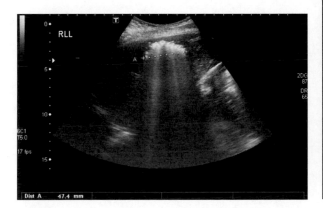

Image 1

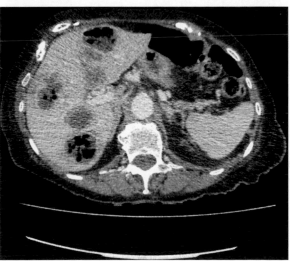

Image 3

R. Joarder et al., *Case Studies in Abdominal and Pelvic Imaging*,
DOI: 10.1007/978-0-85729-366-4_45, © Springer-Verlag London Limited 2011

Answers

1. The ultrasound shows a region of intense reflectivity with posterior acoustic shadowing (Image 4 *black arrow*). This is located within the liver parenchyma and is in keeping with a region of gas.
2. The CT shows multiple abnormalities affecting both lobes of the liver. These are of relatively low attenuation with some patchy peripheral enhancement. Within the centre of some is very low attenuation consistent with air (Image 5 *white arrow*).
3. The radiological features are of hepatic abscesses.

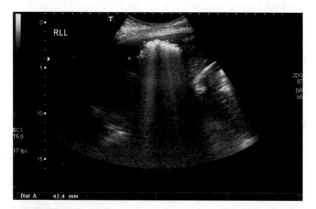

Image 4

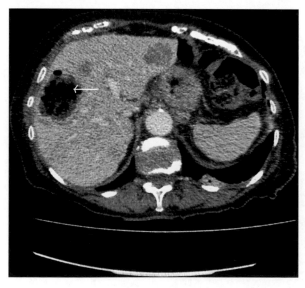

Image 5

A hepatic abscess is a collection of pus within the liver as a result of infection. They are most commonly a result of pyogenic organisms, with about 10% resulting from amoeba and 2% from fungal causes. Gas formation is a feature particularly with *Klebsiella* sp.

Causes include:

Ascending infection from an obstructed biliary tract.
Portal spread from e.g. appendicitis, infective colitis or diverticulitis.
Arterial spread, e.g. endocarditis, urosepsis or IV drug usage.
As a consequence of hepatic infarction.
Direct spread from adjacent infection.
Trauma.

Nearly half are 'cryptogenic' which may be a result of infection of cyst or dead hepatic tissue.

Treatment is with appropriate antibiotics. Drainage, usually radiological, may be required as an adjunct or for microbial identification.

Mortality is high even with treatment. Without treatment hepatic abscess is a fatal condition.

In the given case the clinical history is suspicious for an underlying bowel malignancy. A carcinoembryonic antigen (CEA) measurement was over 1,500 (NR > 5). In general, tumour markers such as CEA are not necessarily diagnostic and may be better used as follow up in a patient known to have disease. However, in this case it further adds to the index of suspicion for malignancy.

Key Points

> Untreated or unrecognised hepatic abscess is a fatal condition.
> Nearly half of cases have no obvious precipitating cause.
> The presence of air within the lesion is an important diagnostic sign.

Further Reading

O'Farrell N, Collins CG, McEntee GP (2010) Pyogenic liver abscesses: Diminished role for operative treatment. Surgeon. Aug;8(4):192-196

A 45-year-old female patient was referred for US-guided liver biopsy prior to commencing therapy for hepatitis C. The US revealed a 5-cm solid hypoechoic mass in segment 6 of the liver.

MRI with dynamic and hepatobiliary phase imaging with gadolinium BOPTA was performed (Image 1, TI axial – unenhanced; Image 2, T2 axial; Image 3, T1 axial – arterial phase contrast enhanced; Image 4, T1 axial – equilibrium phase contrast enhanced; Image 5, T1 axial – hepatobiliary (1 h) phase contrast enhanced).

Questions

1. Describe T1 and T2 signal characteristics of the mass.
2. Describe the contrast enhancement characteristics in the three phases shown.
3. What is the brightly enhancing structure just anteromedial to the mass in Image 5?
4. What is the diagnosis?

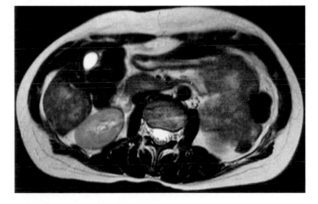

Image 2

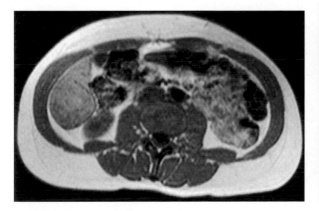

Image 1

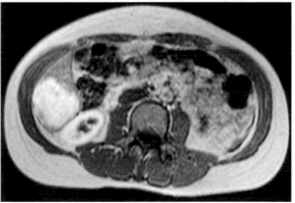

Image 3

R. Joarder et al., *Case Studies in Abdominal and Pelvic Imaging*, DOI: 10.1007/978-0-85729-366-4_46, © Springer-Verlag London Limited 2011

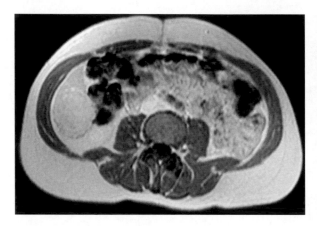

Image 4

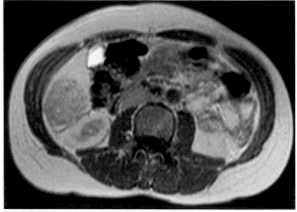

Image 5

Answers

1. Slightly low signal on T1 (*arrow* on Image 6) and slightly high signal on T2 relative to normal liver parenchyma (*arrow* Image 7).
2. Avid arterial phase enhancement (*arrow* Image 8) with less intense enhancement in the equilibrium phase (*arrow* Image 9). Reduced uptake of gadolinium BOPTA, compared to normal hepatic parenchyma, in the hepatobiliary phase (*short arrow* Image 10).
3. The gallbladder (*long arrow* Image 10) – 3% of gadolinium BOPTA is excreted in the bile.
4. Hepatic adenoma.

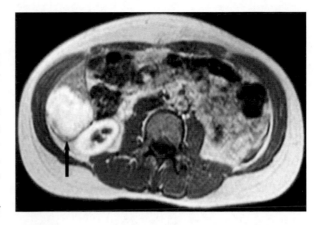

Image 8

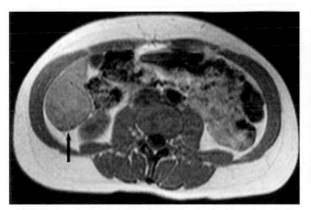

Image 6

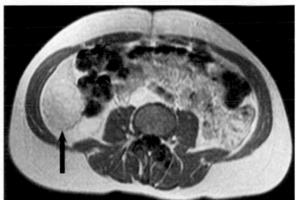

Image 9

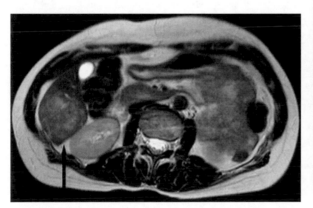

Image 7

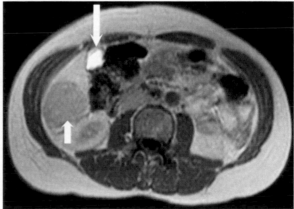

Image 10

This hepatic adenoma was resected because of the risk of haemorrhage and malignant change.

Hepatic adenomas are usually discovered incidentally. These benign hepatic tumours are most common in female patients of reproductive age. Spontaneous haemorrhage – especially during pregnancy is a complication. For this reason large or peripheral lesions in patients wanting to become pregnant may be resected. They have malignant potential.

MRI imaging is often characteristic – low/isointense signal on T1, high/isointense on T2 with strong arterial enhancement and fairly rapid contrast washout during dynamic enhancement with gadolinium. In the hepatobiliary phase of enhancement they show reduced uptake of gadolinium BOPTA compared to normal hepatic parenchyma. Gadolinium BOPTA is used for conventional dynamic enhancement but has a valuable secondary enhancement characteristic – approximately 3% is excreted by hepatocytes into the biliary system. Therefore imaging in the hepatobiliary phase (40–60 min after contrast) will determine whether there are functioning hepatocytes in the lesion – for instance metastases are low signal compared to normal hepatic parenchyma. It is also useful in distinguishing hepatic adenomas (reduced uptake) from focal nodular hyperplasia (FNH) (similar or increased uptake compared to normal hepatic parenchyma – enhancement is increased as bile accumulates in FNH as biliary drainage is impaired) which can otherwise appear identical on MRI [1] (compare to Case 25).

Key Points

> MRI is useful for characterising hepatic lesions.
> Gadolinium BOPTA enhanced MRI is useful for distinguishing hepatic adenomas from FNH.

Reference

1. Grazioli L Morana G, Kirchin MA, et al. (2005) Accurate differentiation of focal nodular hyperplasia from hepatic adenoma at gadobenate dimeglumine-enhanced MR imaging: prospective study. Radiology 236(1):166-77

A 49-year-old female was admitted with a fever and a leucocytosis. There was a past history of open chole-cystectomy, appendicectomy and open abdominal hys-terectomy and oophorectomy. A CT of the abdomen and pelvis was performed (Image 1a and b).

Questions

1. What do Images 1a and b show?
2. Given the history what are the possible diagnoses?

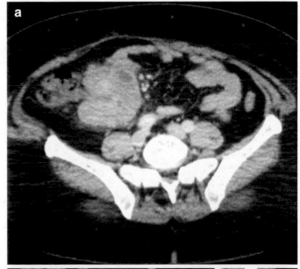

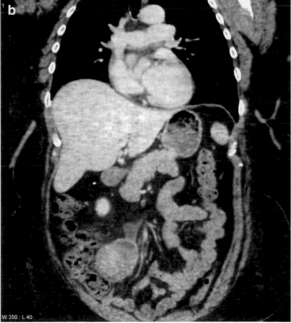

Image 1

R. Joarder et al., *Case Studies in Abdominal and Pelvic Imaging*,
DOI: 10.1007/978-0-85729-366-4_47, © Springer-Verlag London Limited 2011

Answers

1. A large soft tissue mass involving the distal ileum (Images 2a and b).
2. Possible diagnoses would include a small bowel malignancy, such as carcinoid; however, on resection and histological examination it was found to be desmoid fibromatosis.

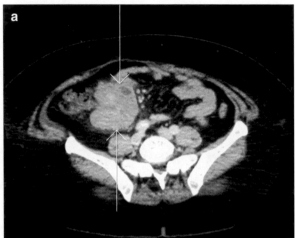

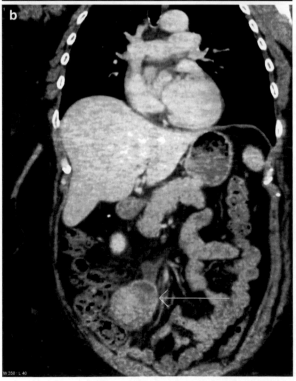

Image 2

Desmoid fibromatosis is a histologically benign tumour known for its aggressive local infiltration and lack of metastatic potential. Complete surgical resection is the treatment of choice.

They are primarily located within the abdominal wall or the abdominal cavity, particularly within the mesentery of the ileum. Patients are often female and there is frequently a history of previous surgery (as in this case). There is also an association with familial polyposis coli.

Patients can be asymptomatic; the most common symptoms are nausea and abdominal pain due to pressure effects. Occasionally, an inflammatory reaction occurs giving, as in our case, a fever and a leucocytosis.

Key Points

> In female patients with previous significant surgical history and an RIF mass, desmoid fibromatosis should be considered.
> Malignancy needs to be considered.
> Complete surgical resection is essential as there is a tendency for local recurrence.

Further Readings

TS Hung et al (2004) Spontaneous Isolated Pedunculated Mesenteric Fibromatosis in a Patient with Acute Abdominal Pain and Persistent Fever.; J Med Sci 24(4):227-230

M Overhaus et al (2003) Desmoid tumours of the abdominal wall: A case report. World J Surg Oncol. 1:11

A 75-year-old woman was seen in out patients with a history of vague abdominal pain and weight loss. She had recently become jaundiced. An MDCT was performed as part of the investigation.

Questions

1. What does the CT show?
2. What is the most likely diagnosis?
3. What treatment options are available?

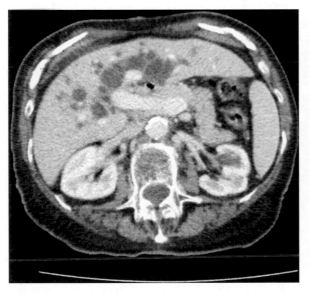

Image 1

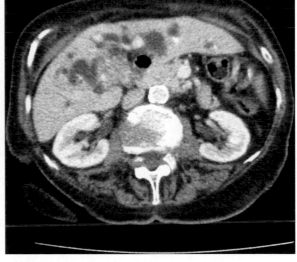

Image 2

R. Joarder et al., *Case Studies in Abdominal and Pelvic Imaging*,
DOI: 10.1007/978-0-85729-366-4_48, © Springer-Verlag London Limited 2011

Answers

1. There is marked intrahepatic biliary dilatation (Image 3 *black arrows*). There is a soft tissue attenuation region at the confluence of the right and left intrahepatic bile ducts. The common bile duct and the pancreatic duct are not dilated (*white arrow*). The pancreas appears normal. Small gall stones are seen.
2. There is an obstructing abnormality at the porta. This is most likely to be a Klatskin tumour, a cholangiocarcinoma at the hilum/bifurcation of the bile ducts.
3. Radical surgery is felt to offer the only possibility of cure. This may be a hepatic resection or orthotropic liver transplantation.

Klatskin described a local adenocarcinoma of the biliary bifurcation as a separate tumour entity in 1965. Only curative resection offers the possibility of long term survival and cure. The trend towards increasingly radical surgery has increased quoted resection rates from 50% to 60% with 5-year survival quoted as 35–45%. The majority of recurrences occur locally and neo-adjuvant and adjuvant therapeutic protocols are becoming increasingly important. These include photodynamic therapy (PDT).

The mainstay of palliative treatment is stenting and PDT may have a role. Radio-/chemotherapy does not seem to offer any benefit.

Other processes may affect the hilum causing biliary obstruction and mimicking a Klatskin tumour. These include malignant processes such as lymphoma. Tuberculosis affecting the hepatic porta has also been reported.

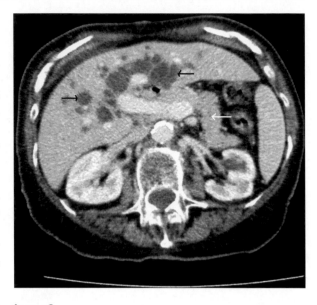

Image 3

Key Points

> Obstruction at the biliary confluence will cause intra-hepatic biliary dilatation with a normal calibre CBD.
> Surgical resection of such tumours is felt to offer the best survival chance.

Further Readings

Hilar cholangiocarcinoma: current management. Ito F, Cho CS, Rikkers LF, Weber SM. Ann Surg. 2009 Aug;250(2):210-8

Witzigmann H, Wiedmann M, Wittekind C, Mössner J, Hauss J. Therapeutical concepts and results for klatskin tumors. Dtsch Arztebl Int. 2008 Feb;105(9):156-61

A 34-year-old patient with a long history of RUQ pain presented with jaundice and fever. US showed dilated intrahepatic ducts and CBD (12 mm), but the cause of the biliary dilation was not shown. An MRCP was performed – Image 1, coronal T2; Image 2, coronal MIP; and Image 3, axial T2.

Questions

1. What does the MRCP show?
2. What should be done next?

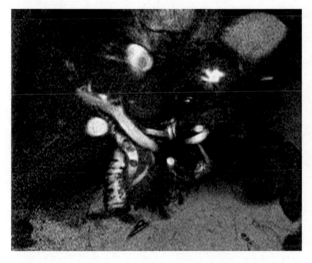

Image 2

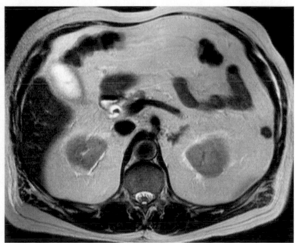

Image 1

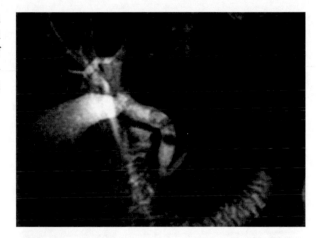

Image 3

R. Joarder et al., *Case Studies in Abdominal and Pelvic Imaging*,
DOI: 10.1007/978-0-85729-366-4_49, © Springer-Verlag London Limited 2011

Answers

1. Rounded low signal (*black*) filling defects (*arrows* Images 4–6) within the high signal (*white*) bile of the dilated distal CBD.
2. ERCP with stone removal. ERCP (Image 7) – CBD stone (*arrow*).

US is accurate in the detection of gallstones in the gall-bladder, but much less so for choledocholithiasis. If choledocholithiasis is suspected – for instance history

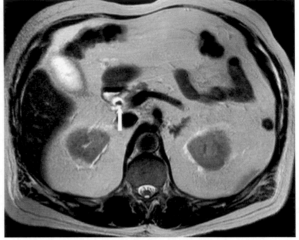

Image 6

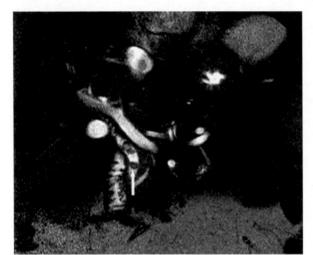

Image 4

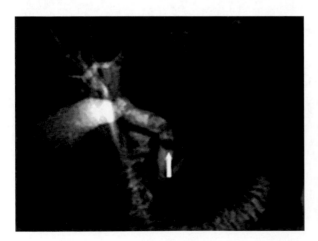

Image 5

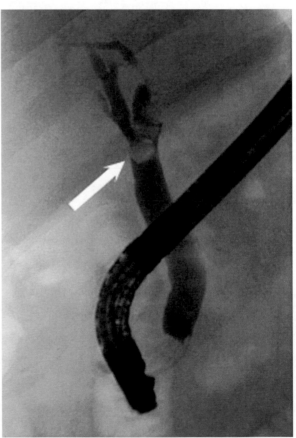

Image 7

of gallstones or cholecystectomy and subsequent jaundice or right upper quadrant pain and jaundice – US may be performed, but mainly to detect biliary dilatation. Sometimes US may detect bile duct stones, but if there is biliary dilatation and stones are suspected, MRCP is usually performed. This is accurate for the detection of gallstones in both the gallbladder and bile duct. Probably not as accurate as ERCP or EUS (particularly in large patients or those unable to hold their breath) but has the advantage of being non-invasive and non-ionising radiation.

Key Points

> US is accurate for detection of gallstones in the gallbladder, but much less so for choledocholithiasis.

> If choledocholithiasis is suspected, MRCP is the preferred investigation particularly if US has detected biliary dilatation but no bile duct stones.

A 17-year-old female with a 1-month history of RIF pain, on contraceptive implant. An US (Images 1a and b) and an MRI (Images 2a, b and 3a, b) of the pelvis were performed.

Questions

1. What do Images 1a and b of the RIF show?
2. What is the sequence in Images 2a and b and what do they show?
3. What are the sequences in Images 3a and b and what do they show?
4. What is the most likely diagnosis?

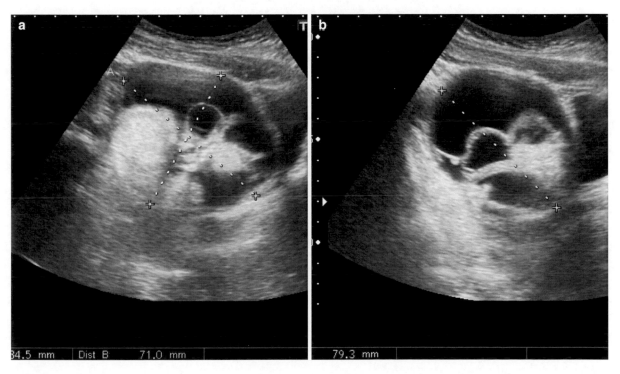

Image 1

R. Joarder et al., *Case Studies in Abdominal and Pelvic Imaging*,
DOI: 10.1007/978-0-85729-366-4_50, © Springer-Verlag London Limited 2011

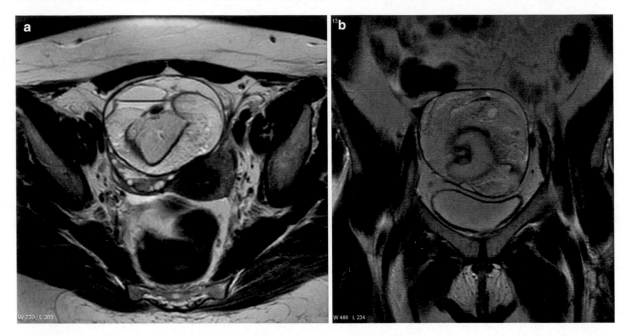

Image 2

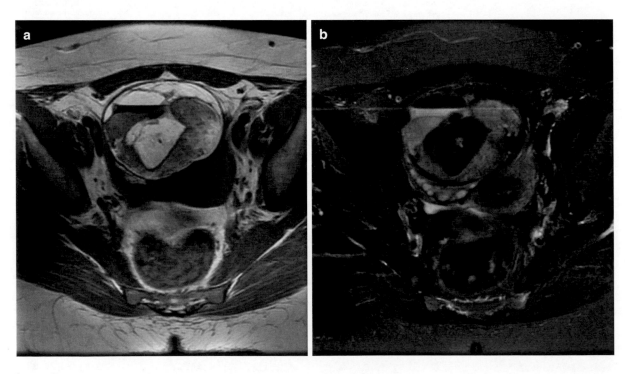

Image 3

Answers

1. A solid cystic mass. The solid area is particularly echogenic.
2. Axial and coronal T2 scans. These confirm a heterogeneous mass with predominantly high signal throughout the lesion but low signal septations. There is the suggestion of a fluid level anteriorly on the right within the lesion.
3. Axial T1 and T2 fat saturated scans. These show that the central high signal area and the more anterior aspect of the fluid level remain high signal on T1 imaging and become low signal on T2 fat saturated images indicating that these are areas of fat. The areas of high signal surrounding the central fat and the more posterior fluid are low signal on T1 and high signal on T2 fat saturated images indicating fluid. The fluid level is a fat fluid level with the fat floating.
4. Dermoid cyst.

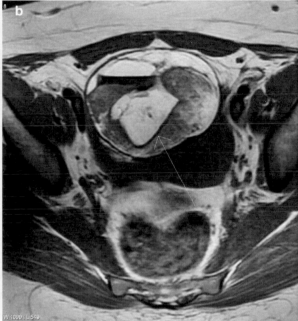

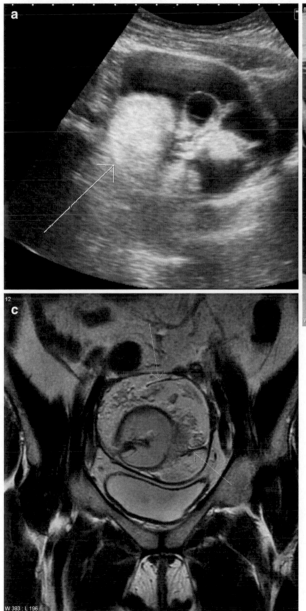

Image 4

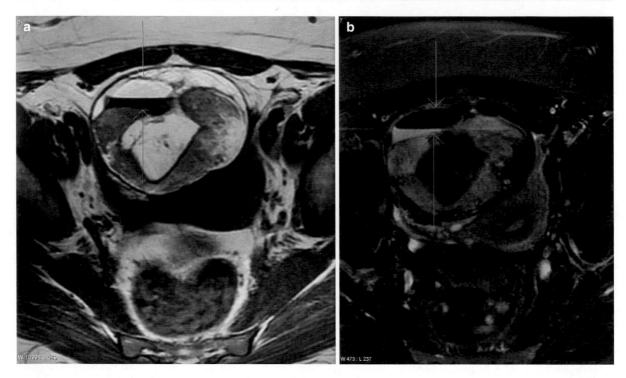

Image 5

Ovarian dermoid cysts, also known as mature cystic teratomas, have a variety of appearances. The three most common features are of a cystic lesion with a dense tubercle (Rokitansky nodule) (Image 4a) which projects into the cystic lumen, a diffusely echogenic mass on US, high signal on T1 and T2 imaging representing fatty material (Image 4b) and thin bands seen on US as septations and on MR as low signal thin structures caused by hair within the cyst image (Image 4c). Fat fluid levels are also frequently seen as in this case (Images 5a and b).

Key Points

> Features of dermoid cysts include: cystic areas, fatty tissue, nodules and septations.
> Fat fluid levels can also be seen.

Further Reading

Eric K Outwater et al (2001) Ovarian Teratomas: tumour types and imaging characteristics; Radiographics. 21 :475-490

An 82-year-old man presented to the Emergency Department complaining of abdominal pain and distension.

He had non-insulin dependant diabetes and a history of atrial fibrillation for which he took warfarin.

On examination his abdomen was generally tender and distended. He had evidence of biventricular failure.

An AXR was obtained.

Questions

1. What does the abdominal film show?
2. What are the possible causes and what is the most likely diagnosis?
3. What further investigations should be performed?
4. What examination has been performed and what does it show?
5. What further investigation is required?
6. What are the treatment options?

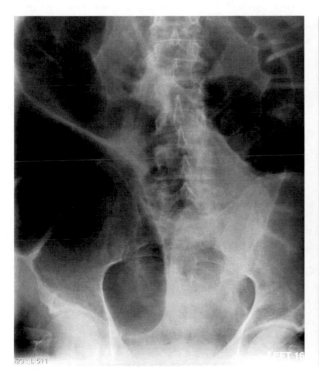

Image 1

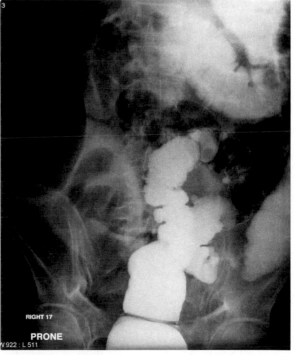

Image 2 Contrast study

R. Joarder et al., *Case Studies in Abdominal and Pelvic Imaging*, DOI: 10.1007/978-0-85729-366-4_51, © Springer-Verlag London Limited 2011

Answers

1. The AXR shows significant dilatation of large bowel with the caecum measuring maximally 16 cm (Image 3 *arrows*). Even though the lateral wall of the abdomen has not been visualised, it possible to follow bowel through ascending colon, transverse and descending colon to mid/lower sigmoid where there is a change in calibre. No gas is seen in the rectum. No evidence of small bowel dilatation is seen. The features are of distal large bowel obstruction.

2. In an adult the broad categories of differential diagnosis are:
   i.   Luminal obstruction, e.g. faecal impaction, gall stone in narrowed sigmoid
   ii. Bowel wall lesion – malignant; inflammatory, e.g. colitis or diverticulitis; infectious or wall haematoma
   iii. Extrinsic – mass compression, e.g. endometriosis, pelvic mass/abscess; or severe constriction, e.g. volvulus

   The most common causes are, in order, malignancy, sigmoid diverticulitis and volvulus.

3. Delineation of the bowel is required. This can be done with water soluble contrast enema, possibly followed by CT.

4. The image is a single view from a water soluble contrast enema. The investigation shows a typical 'apple core' type lesion in the sigmoid consistent with a malignancy (Image 4).

5. Full staging of the tumour is required by CT of the chest abdomen and pelvis. Given the pattern of obstruction on plain film and enema findings, the diagnosis of malignancy is secure radiologically. Depending on circumstance, direct visualisation and biopsy may be thought necessary prior to treatment.

6. The obstruction needs to be relieved. This could be by surgical resection of the tumour. In this case the patient was not thought fit for surgery immediately and a colonic stent was inserted as a bridge to surgery.

A water soluble contrast enema is preferred to barium in the acute event. Leakage of barium into the abdominal cavity can cause a marked inflammatory reaction and so barium should be avoided if there is a possibility of perforation/leakage or if the patient will undergo surgery in a very short time frame.

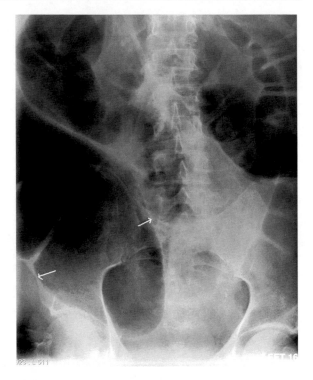

Image 3

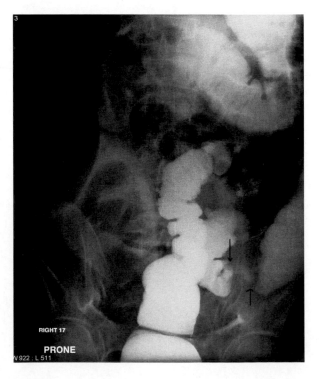

Image 4

Endoscopically inserted colonic stents can be used to relieve obstruction. They may be used as a short-term bridge to definitive surgical treatment or a palliative measure if surgery is not thought appropriate.

Complications include stent migration, blockage and fistulation in to adjacent organs.

Key Points

> Malignancy is the most common cause of large bowel obstruction in adults.
> Water soluble media should be used in preference to barium if there is a risk of perforation or imminent surgery.
> Endoscopic or radiologically inserted colonic stents can be used as a bridge to surgery or as a palliative measure.

Further Reading

Athreya S, Mossa J, Urguhart G et al (2006) Colorectal stenting for colonic obstruction: The indications, complications, effectiveness and outcome—5-Year review. Eur J Radiology 60 (1): 91-94
Dharmadhikari R, Nice C (2007) Complications of colonic stenting: a pictorial review. Abdom Imaging 33(3):278-84

A 50-year-old male presented with non-specific central abdominal pain. Appetite and weight were stable and all blood test normal. An MDCT was performed (Image 1). A CT-guided adrenal biopsy was performed and no treatment was given but a follow-up CT was performed 3 months later (Image 2).

Questions

1. Comment on the abnormality – location and density.
2. What has happened to the abnormality on the follow-up MDCT?
3. What is the diagnosis?

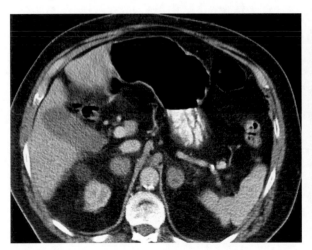

Image 1

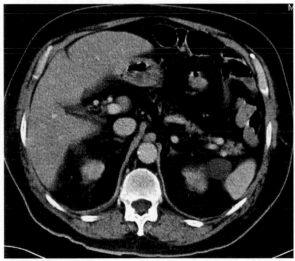

Image 2

R. Joarder et al., *Case Studies in Abdominal and Pelvic Imaging*,
DOI: 10.1007/978-0-85729-366-4_52, © Springer-Verlag London Limited 2011

Answers

1. There are small bilateral high density adrenal masses (*arrows* Image 3).
2. The adrenal glands now appear normal (*arrows* Image 4).
3. Bilateral adrenal haemorrhage.

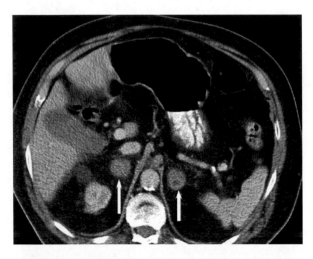

Image 3

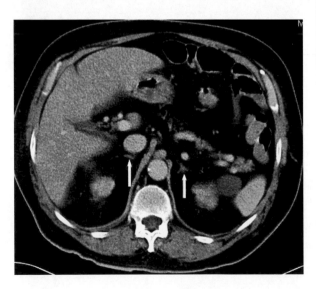

Image 4

Spontaneous adrenal haemorrhage is a rare and heterogenous condition. It is associated with several clinical situations including severe stress/sepsis, post-operative period, antiphospholipid antibody syndrome and anticoagulation. In these scenarios adrenal haemorrhage can lead to adrenal failure, multi-organ failure and death.

Adrenal haemorrhage is often associated with adrenal failure and this sought by measuring serum cortisol. Biochemical testing is complimented by imaging – the gold standard is MDCT.

However adrenal haemorrhage may be asymptomatic and discovered incidentally on imaging. In this scenario the prognosis is good and the haemorrhage usually resolves. Adrenal function should be monitored to detect adrenal failure. In cases of spontaneous incidental adrenal haemorrhage, particularly bilateral, antiphospholipid antibody syndrome should be excluded.

Key Points

> Spontaneous adrenal haemorrhage is rare in adults.
> It is associated with various underlying conditions and can lead to adrenal failure and death.
> However, incidentally discovered adrenal haemorrhage has a good prognosis.

Further Reading

Vella A, Todd B, Nippoldt MD, et al. (2001) Adrenal haemorrhage: A 25-year experience at the Mayo Clinic. Mayo Clin Proc 76:161-168

An 80-year-old female, 5 days post-laparoscopic hysterectomy for fibroids, developed vomiting and abdominal pain. An AXR (Image 1) and a CT of the abdomen and pelvis (Images 2a and b) were performed.

Questions

1. What does the AXR show?
2. What is the cause demonstrated on CT?
3. What reason relating to the recent surgery can you think of?

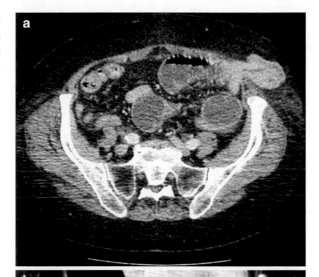

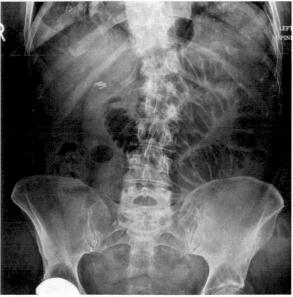

Image 1

Image 2

R. Joarder et al., *Case Studies in Abdominal and Pelvic Imaging*,
DOI: 10.1007/978-0-85729-366-4_53, © Springer-Verlag London Limited 2011

Answers

1. Mid small bowel obstruction.
2. Spigelian hernia in the left abdominal wall (Images 3a and b).
3. Small bowel had herniated through a 5-mm laparoscopy port site.

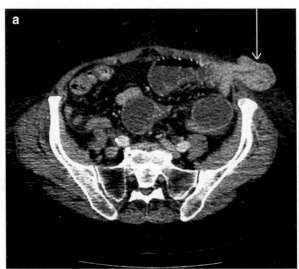

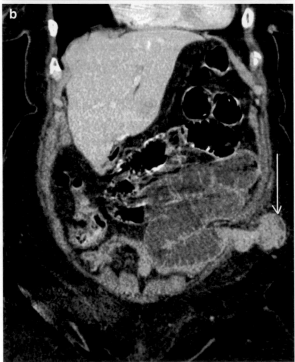

Image 3

The AXR shows significant dilatation of the proximal small bowel with an abrupt cut off. The appearances were not consistent with an ileus as had been suspected clinically.

The CT shows a loop of proximal ileum herniating through the anterior abdominal wall within the left lower quadrant corresponding to a 5-mm laparoscopy port site.

These types of hernias complicating abdominal surgery have an increased incidence in laparoscopic surgery using large trocars.

Key Points

> If only part of the small bowel is dilated it is likely to be due to obstruction rather than an ileus.
> An ileus would usually cause distension of the entire small and large bowel.
> Be aware of this potential complication in patients with abdominal pain following laparoscopic surgery.
> Prompt diagnosis of acute bowel hernia causing obstruction is important to avoid ischaemia at the site of obstruction.

Further Reading

Gill F, and McLucas B. (1996) Spigelian hernia in laparoscopic surgery. Minimally Invasive Therapy and Allied Technologies, 5(6):517-520

An 87-year-old man presented to the Emergency Department with a short history of abdominal pain. He was hypotensive at 80/40.

A CT of the abdomen and pelvis was performed.

Questions

1. What are the CT findings?
2. What is the diagnosis?
3. Is there evidence of acute bleeding?
4. What are the treatment options?

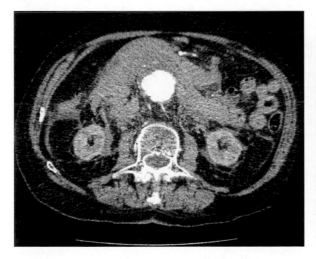

Image 1

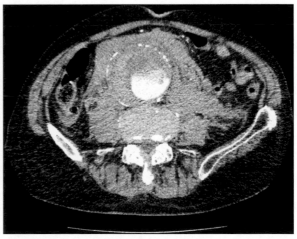

Image 2

Answers

1. The CT shows aneurysmal dilatation of the infra-renal abdominal aorta. Maximum diameter is 8 cm. There is a well-defined lumen with some ill-defined higher attenuation in the region expected to be thrombus (Image 3 *white X*). The calcified wall is seen peripherally (Image 3 *arrows*). There is super added soft tissue anterior and lateral to the aorta (Image 4 *white arrow*). This is consistent with recent extramural haemorrhage.
2. The diagnosis is of a leaking abdominal aortic aneurysm.
3. There is no evidence of active current contrast extravasation. The linear high attenuation seen posterior to the aorta is within a lumbar vessel. There is evidence of extensive recent contained leak.
4. Treatment involves surgical repair or endovascular stent grafting.

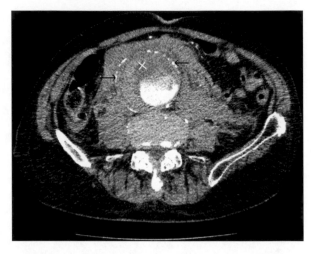

Image 3

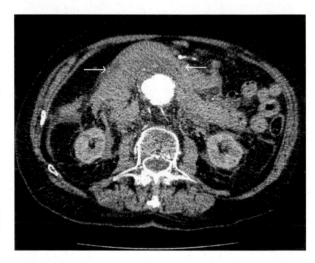

Image 4

Key Points

> Leaking aortic aneurysm is a serious surgical emergency with high morbidity.
> Pre-operative diagnosis with CT is quick and simple; although undue delay waiting for CT should be avoided.

A 59-year-old male presented with upper abdominal pain, weight loss and jaundice.

LFTs were abnormal with elevated bilirubin and alkaline phosphatase.

US demonstrated a dilated biliary tree but no gall-stones in the gallbladder.

MDCT with oral contrast was performed (Image 1).

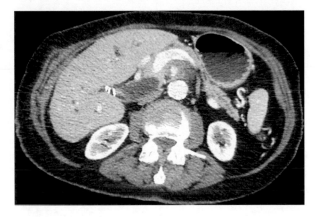

Image 1

Questions

1. Identify and describe the CBD.
2. Identify the SMA and describe the area around the SMA.

Answers

1. The CBD is dilated (*long arrow* Image 2)
2. The SMA is encircled by soft tissue (*short arrow* Image 2). This is due to malignant tissue from locally invasive carcinoma of the pancreas. The SMA should be surrounded by low attenuation fat (*arrow* Image 3).

Pancreatic carcinoma is common and usually has a dismal prognosis as the tumour is often locally invasive with metastatic disease at presentation. MDCT is accurate in the staging of pancreatic carcinoma.

The size of the tumour can be accurately measured (although can be difficult to see particularly if only imaged in portal venous phase rather than the earlier pancreatic phase).

Invasion of adjacent structure, particularly mesenteric vessels – SMA, SMV and gastroduodenal vessels – is reliably assessed.

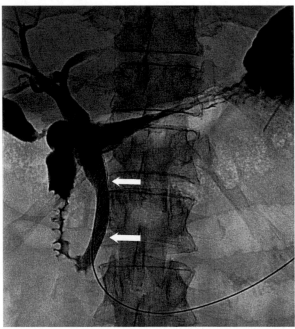

Image 4

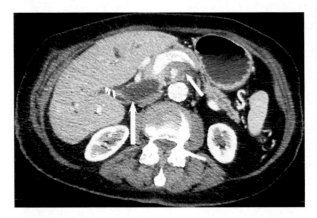

Image 2

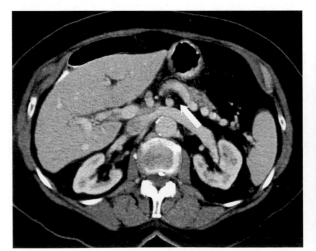

Image 3

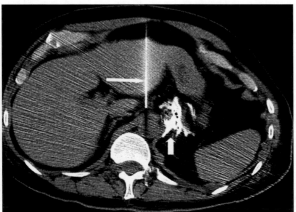

Image 5

IR techniques have a role to play in palliation, i.e. if ERCP or endoscopic duodenal stent insertion are unsuccessful both can be achieved by IR (Image 4 – percutaneous radiological insertion of metallic biliary stent – *arrows*). It also has a role to play in pain relief. If narcotic analgesia is ineffective or associated with unacceptable side effects CT-guided destruction of the coeliac plexus with alcohol can provide good pain control (Image 5 CT-guided neurolysis of coeliac plexus – alcohol mixed with dilute contrast [*short arrow*] has been injected around the left side of the coeliac plexus around the coeliac trunk and the needle has been re-inserted through the liver to the right side to ensure complete ablation – *long arrow*).

Key Points

> CT is accurate for staging carcinoma of the pancreas.
> IR can be useful in relief of biliary obstruction, duodenal obstruction and pain.

A 48-year-old multiparous woman presented with vaginal discomfort, dyspareunia, nocturia and mild stress incontinence. On examination there was a lump visible at the introitus arising from the anterior wall of the vagina. Axial T2 (Image 1), axial T1 (Image 2) and sagittal T2 (Image 3) MRIs were performed.

Questions

1. What do the three MR images show?
2. What are the possible most likely diagnoses?

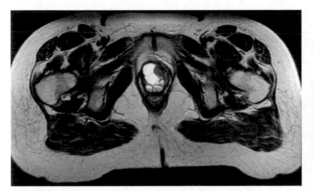

Image 1

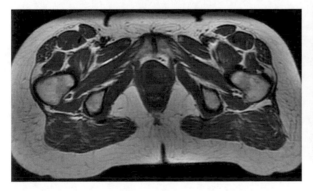

Image 2

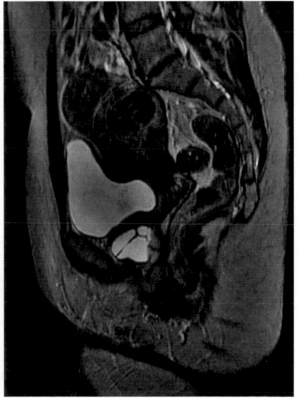

Image 3

Answers

1. The MRI shows a complex, partly septated cystic mass (*vertical arrow* Image 4) displacing the vagina posteriorly and surrounding the urethra (*horizontal arrow* Image 4) on the right. The urethra is displaced to the left; there is no obvious communication with the urethra. Layering of lower signal material is seen posteriorly (Image 5) but no evidence of haemorrhage.

2. Possible diagnoses include a periurethral cyst or a walled-off urethral diverticulum.

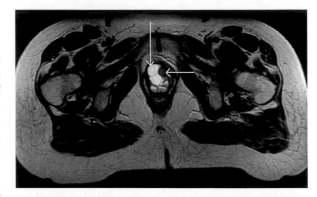

Image 4

At surgery there was an inflamed cystic structure found adherent to the urethra. No communication could be demonstrated between the urethra and the mass using methylene blue injected per urethra. However histologically the resected specimen demonstrated transitional cell epithelium and therefore more in keeping with a urethral diverticulum (presumably walled off secondary to inflammation).

Key Point

> Urethral diverticula can be walled off making them difficult to diagnose at MRI and easy to confuse with urethral cysts.

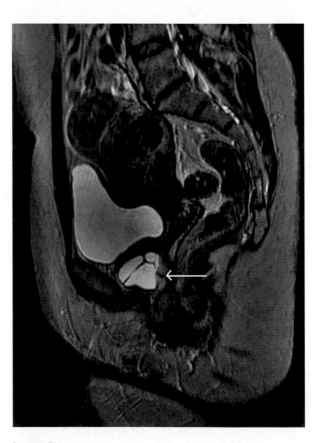

Image 5

A 78-year-old woman had an endovascular repair (EVAR) of an infra-renal abdominal aortic aneurysm.

Post-procedure ultrasound and MDCT were performed.

Questions

1. What do the US and CT show?
2. What is the treatment?
3. What does the image show?
4. How could this be managed?

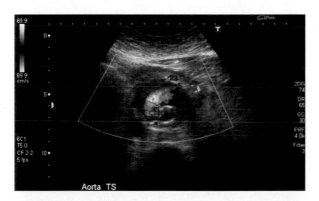

Image 1 US

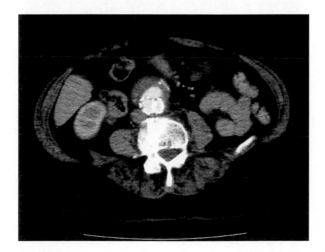

Image 2 CT

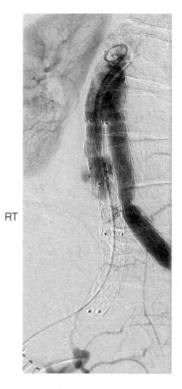

Image 3 An intra-procedural image.

R. Joarder et al., *Case Studies in Abdominal and Pelvic Imaging*,
DOI: 10.1007/978-0-85729-366-4_57, © Springer-Verlag London Limited 2011

Answers

1. The US shows swirling arterial flow within the aneurysm sac. The CT shows the two iliac limbs of the EVAR. There is extravasation of contrast from the device which appears to originate from the right limb (Image 4 *white arrow*). The findings are of a type III endoleak.
2. Treatment is by further stent graft insertion to seal the leak.
3. There is good flow in the left limb of the device. There is no flow in the right limb (Image 5 *long black arrow*), which has been used as the access route for the catheter (*short black arrow*). The features are of thrombus in the right limb. It also shows the endoleak from the right limb (*white arrow*).
4. In this case a balloon occlusion device was used as an embolectomy catheter.

Endovascular stent graft (EVAR) placement is an increasingly popular treatment option for abdominal aortic aneurysms (AAA) avoiding open surgery. Lower rates of complication, 30 days mortality and hospital stay are quoted. The procedure is however not without complication. These include in order of frequency persistent arterial flow within the aneurysm, graft thrombosis, migration and kinking, peripheral embolisation and aortic dissection.

Persistent arterial flow in the aneurysm sac is termed endoleak. Reported incidence varies from 3% to 40%; the majority discovered within 30 days of procedure. Classification is based on the source of communication, with type II the most common.

Type I – flow around distal or proximal attachment sites.

Type II – retrograde flow from aortic branches.

Type III – graft defect or malfunction.

Type IV – graft porosity.

Continued expansion of the aneurysm sac without demonstrable leak is termed endotension and is classified by some as type V.

Up to 12% of patients require additional procedures post-EVAR. Type I and III leaks can be treated with extender cuff insertion; conversion to open operation may be required. Treatment options for type II include catheter embolisation or laparoscopic vessel ligation.

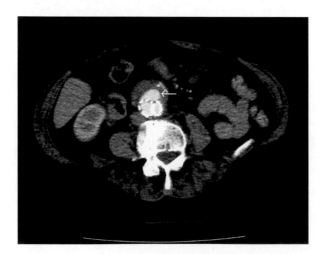

Image 4

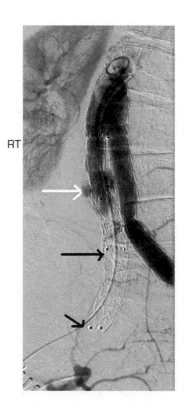

Image 5

Further Readings

Corrie M, Feurer I, Becker S, et al (2004) Endoleak Following Endovascular Abdominal Aortic Aneurysm Repair: Implications for Duration of Screening. Annals of Surgery 239: 800-807

Tolia A, Landis R, Lamparello P, Rosen R, Macari M (2005) Type II Endoleaks after Endovascular Repair of Abdominal Aortic Aneurysms: Natural History. Radiology 235:683-686

A 40 year-old-man who had previously undergone ileal conduit formation presented with sudden onset of generalised, severe abdominal pain. On examination there was abdominal tenderness and no bowel sounds. The patient was tachycardic and hypotensive. Plain films were poor quality due to patient's large size but were thought to show small bowel dilation. An MDCT of the abdomen was performed (Image 1, axial through the liver; Images 2 and 3 axial, through mid-abdomen; and Image 4, coronal abdomen).

Questions

1. Describe the appearance of the liver. What is the cause?
2. Describe the appearance of the small bowel.
3. What is the diagnosis and treatment?
4. What is the congenital abnormality that led to ileal conduit formation?

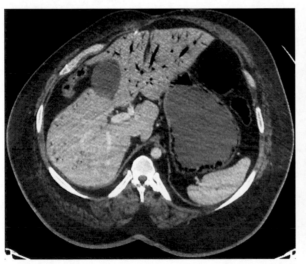

Image 1

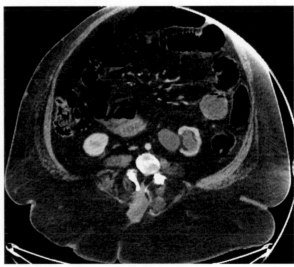

Image 2

R. Joarder et al., *Case Studies in Abdominal and Pelvic Imaging*,
DOI: 10.1007/978-0-85729-366-4_58, © Springer-Verlag London Limited 2011

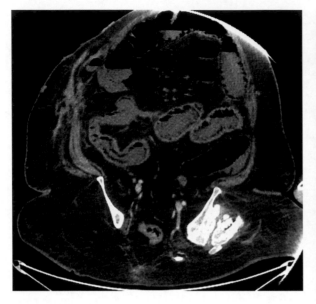

Image 3

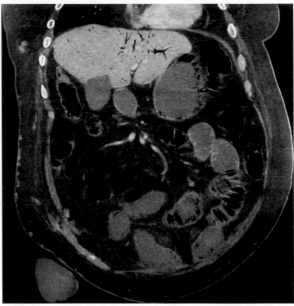

Image 4

Answers

1. There is branching linear air density in the liver predominantly in the left lobe and periphery of the right lobe characteristic of portal vein gas (*arrows* Image 5).
2. There is air within the wall of the small bowel – pneumatosis intestinalis (*arrows* Image 7). There is also some linear air density in the mesentery due to gas in branches of the superior mesenteric vein (*arrow* Image 8).

3. Small bowel ischaemia causing portomesenteric gas. Surgery is mandatory
4. There is spina bifida with a meningocoele (*arrow* Image 6).

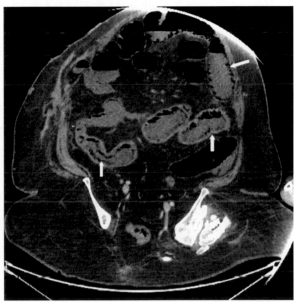

Image 7

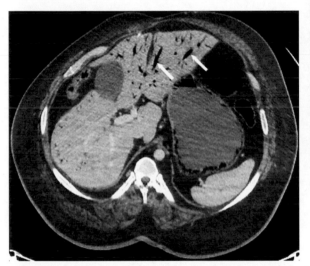

Image 5

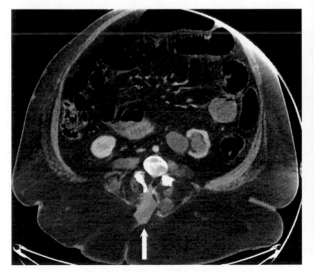

Image 6

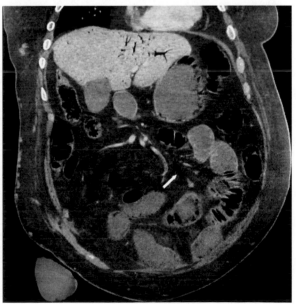

Image 8

The patient underwent laparotomy which confirmed extensive small bowel necrosis requiring resection. The patient died of multi-organ failure several days later.

When intestinal pneumatosis is detected on AXR it is associated with bowel infarction and a very poor prognosis. Its significance when detected on CT is different. Fifty percent of cases are associated with bowel ischaemia, but the other 50% are associated with a variety of conditions including intestinal obstruction, cancer, volvulus, ulcer, hernia, trauma, Crohn's disease, diverticulitis and iatrogenic causes. The overall mortality is 30%. On CT bubbles of gas are seen in the bowel wall.

Portomesenteric gas is most frequently due to bowel ischaemia but there are many causes and 15% are idiopathic.

CT is more sensitive than plain abdominal X-rays in the detection of portomesenteric gas. CT features are linear branching areas of air density peripherally in the liver, especially the left lobe. Gas in the larger mesenteric veins is linear air density along the course of the mesenteric veins – usually also containing contrast – passing between the mesenteric border of the bowel towards the liver.

Seventy percent of patients with both intestinal pneumatosis and portomesenteric vein have intestinal ischaemia and a mortality of 50%.

Key Points

> Portomesentric vein gas and have characteristic appearance on CT.
> The commonest cause of portomesenteric vein gas and intestinal pneumatosis is bowel ischaemia for which surgery is mandatory.

Further Readings

Lassandro F, di Santo Stefano ML, Maria Porto A, et al (2010) Intestinal pneumatosis: diagnostic and prognostic value. Emerg Radiol April 15 (Epub ahead of print)
Sebastia S, Quiroga S, Espin E, et al. (2000) Portomesenteric vein gas: pathologic mechanisms, CT findings and prognosis. Radiographics 20(5):1213-24

Case 59

A 38-year-old female presented with dyspareunia and irregular periods. A pelvic US (Image 1) followed by sagittal T2 (Image 2a) axial T2 (Image 2b) and axial T1 (Image 2c) MRI scans.

Questions

1. What does Image 1 show?
2. What do Images 2a–c show?
3. What is the likely diagnosis?

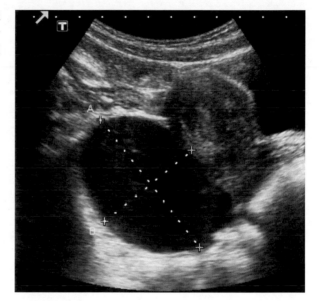

Image 1

R. Joarder et al., *Case Studies in Abdominal and Pelvic Imaging*,
DOI: 10.1007/978-0-85729-366-4_59, © Springer-Verlag London Limited 2011

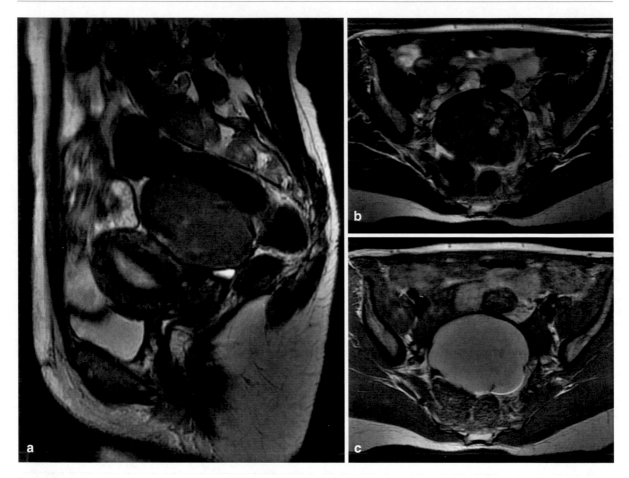

Image 2

Answers

1. There is a predominantly hypoechoic mass (*vertical arrow* Image 3) posterior to the uterus (*horizontal arrow* Image 3) which has some echoes within it.
2. On MRI the mass (*vertical arrow* Image 4a) is confirmed to be posterior to the uterus (*horizontal arrow* Image 4a). It is predominantly low signal on T2 with patchy areas of increased signal seen on the axial T2 scan (*arrows* Image 4b) and of high signal throughout on T1 (*arrows* Image 4c). These signal characteristics are indicative of blood. Given the low signal on T2 this suggests that the bleed is in the early subacute phase.
3. Endometriosis, the mass represents an endometrioma of the right ovary.

The MRI appearances of a subacute haematoma are of low signal on T2 and high signal on T1 due to the presence of *intra*cellular methaemaglobin. Whilst a T1 fat saturated scan would be useful to confirm the appearances, the signal characteristics on T2 are not of fat. If the haematoma were a little older the cyst would appear as high signal on both T1 and T2 due to *extra*cellular methaemaglobin and more difficult to differentiate from fat; if this were the case, a fat saturated scan would be necessary.

Endometriosis is characterized by the presence of ectopic endometrial tissue outside the uterus most commonly within the pelvis involving the ovaries, fallopian tubes, broad and round ligaments, cervix, vagina and pouch of Douglas. It tends to occur in women of reproductive age. Other sites include the gastrointestinal tract and urinary tract. Symptoms, as in the case above, often include dyspareunia and irregular bleeding, but also dysmenorrhoea and pelvic pain.

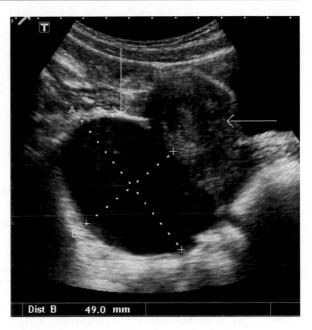

Image 3

The US appearances of endometrioma can vary widely; however diffuse internal echoes occur in 95% of lesions. The MRI appearances are generally of ovarian masses with evidence of haemorrhage.

Laparoscopy is the gold standard for diagnosis of endometriosis. US and MRI have sensitivities of 83% and 90% and specificities of 98% and 98%, respectively, for diagnosing endometrioma. It is very difficult to detect an implant outside the ovaries using US; MRI also has a low sensitivity of 27% on standard T1 and T2 sequences. The sensitivity improves to 61% if fat saturated T1 sequences are used to identify haemorrhage.

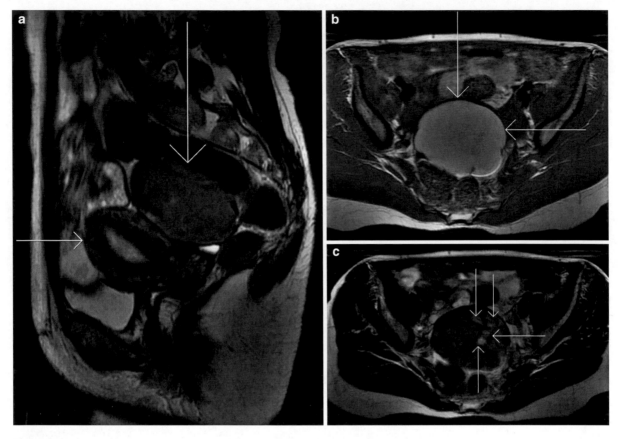

Image 4

Further Reading

Umaria N, Olliff JF (2001) Imaging features of pelvic endometriosis. British Journal of Radiology 74: 556-562

Key Points

> On US if an ovarian cyst (unilateral or bilat-
  eral) has internal echoes in a woman of reproductive age, consider endometrioma.
> On MRI if the cyst has high signal on T1 +/– T2,
  consider endometrioma.
> If the MRI is to attempt to identify endometrial
  implants outside the ovaries, always perform a
  fat-saturated T1 sequence.

A 58-year-old man was seen in outpatients complaining of pain and swelling in the right groin. Clinical examination showed no evidence of a hernia. As part of the investigation an X-ray of the pelvis and MRI of the hips were performed.

Questions

1. What abnormality does the plain film show?
2. What abnormalities does the MRI show?
3. What is the most likely underlying diagnosis and what additional investigations are required?

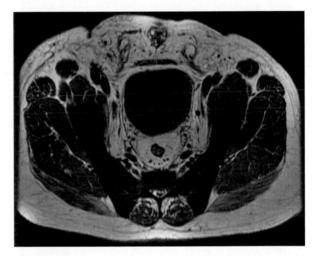

Image 2

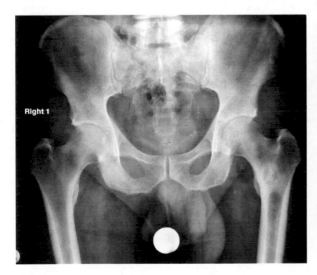

Image 1

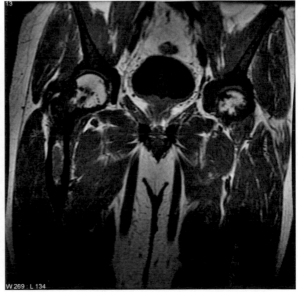

Image 3

R. Joarder et al., *Case Studies in Abdominal and Pelvic Imaging*,
DOI: 10.1007/978-0-85729-366-4_60, © Springer-Verlag London Limited 2011

Answers

1. The plain film of the hips shows several areas of ill defined sclerosis of the bones. This is most noticeable in the region of the left SI joint, the lower lumber spine and the intertrochanteric region of the left femur (Image 4).
2. The MRI images given are of T1 weighting. Fat is high signal and fluid dark.

   There is extensive abnormal low signal in the bone marrow of the pelvis (Image 5). At this age bone marrow signal should be bright on T1 reflecting fatty content. The low signal represents bone marrow infiltration.
3. There is evidence of diffuse bone infiltration by metastatic disease. Given the sclerotic appearance on plain film and the gender of the patient the most likely underlying diagnosis is of prostate cancer.

Further investigation with a prostate specific antigen (PSA) and an isotope bone scan is needed. In this case the PSA was over 300 (normal range up to 4). The bone scan confirmed the presence of extensive bone lesions.

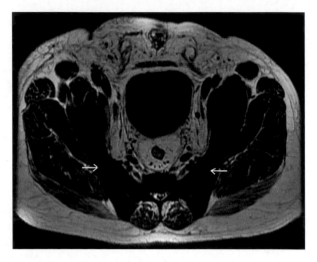

Image 5

Given the high PSA and evidence of disseminated disease on radiology, a clinical diagnosis of prostate cancer can be made and a biopsy of the gland is not required.

Key Points

› Prostate cancer is common and may present late with established metastatic disease.
› Sclerotic bone metastases are typical.
› Radionuclide imaging is very useful in assessing the extent of bone disease.

Further Readings

Ibrahim T, Flamini E, Mercatali L, Sacanna E, Serra P, Amadori D. (2010). Pathogenesis of osteoblastic bone metastases from prostate cancer. Cancer. 116(6):1406-18.

Persec Z, Persec J, Sović T, Romic Z, Bosnar Herak M, Hrgovic Z. (2010) Metastatic prostate cancer in an asymptomatic patient with an initial prostate-specific antigen (PSA) serum concentration of 21,380 ng/ml. Onkologie.33(3):110-2.

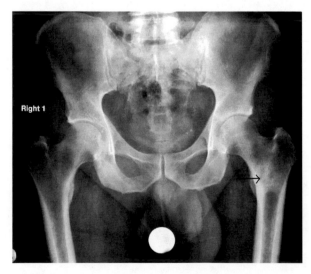

Right 1

Image 4

A 24-year-old male with a 10-year history of ulcerative colitis gave a history of episodes of RUQ pain and fevers. On examination he was jaundiced. His LFTS were deranged with an obstructive pattern. Imaging was requested (Image 1).

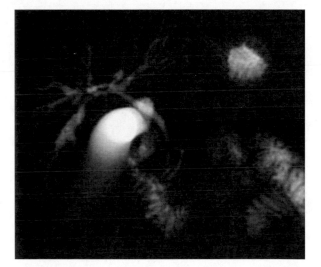

Image 1

Questions

1. What is the examination?
2. Comment on the gallbladder, common bile duct and intra-hepatic ducts.
3. What is the diagnosis?

R. Joarder et al., *Case Studies in Abdominal and Pelvic Imaging*,
DOI: 10.1007/978-0-85729-366-4_61, © Springer-Verlag London Limited 2011

Answers

1. MRCP.
2. The gallbladder appears normal with no stones (*short arrow* Image 2). The common bile duct is of irregular calibre – with mild narrowing proximally and distally (*long arrows* Image 2). The intra-hepatic bile ducts show areas of both narrowing and dilatation with the suggestion of low signal filling defects in the dilated segment 5/8 duct (*medium arrow* Image 2) – possibly stones/debris.
3. Primary sclerosing cholangitis (PSC).

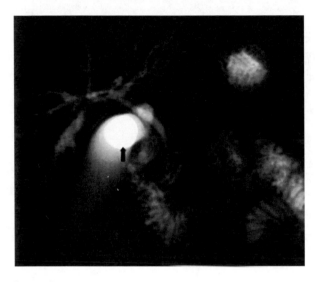

Image 2

Primary sclerosing cholangitis is an autoimmune disease causing chronic cholestatis leading to biliary cirrhosis. The imaging features ERCP and MRCP are typical – irregular stenoses and dilations of the intra- and extra-hepatic bile ducts. As in this case, stones or debris can form in the dilated segments. Classical cases as above are straightforward, but the images can be difficult to interpret in early disease.

Seventy percent of patients with PSC have ulcerative colitis and approximately 5% of patients with UC have PSC. There is no specific treatment. Liver transplantation may be necessary and has a good survival rate.

In patients with PSC there is a high risk of cholangiocarcinoma – screening with MRCP is sometimes advocated but unproven. Once cholangiocarcinoma has developed there is a poor prognosis.

Key Points

> PSC has typical MRCP/ERCP features.
> Early PSC can be difficult to detect on imaging.
> There is a high risk of developing cholangiocarcinoma.

Further Reading

Weismuller TJ, Wedemeyer J, Kubicka S, et al. (2008) The challenges in primary sclerosing cholangitis – aetiopathogenesis, autoimmunity, management and malignancy. J Hepatol 48(1):38-57

A 26-year-old female admitted with acute abdominal pain, vomiting and pyrexia one week after emergency caesarean section for failed induction of labour.

On examination, she was tachycardic, pyrexial and had generalised abdominal discomfort. Her WBC and ESR were raised. An US of the upper abdomen (Images 1a and b) and a CXR (Image 2) were performed.

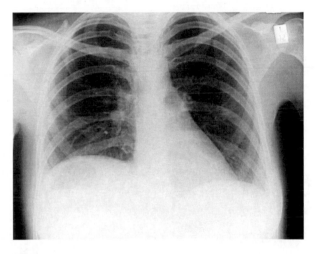

Image 2

Questions

1. What do Images 1a and b show?
2. What does Image 2 show?
3. What is the likely cause for the patient's symptoms?

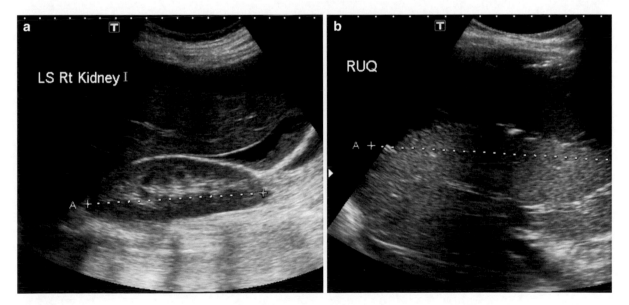

Image 1

R. Joarder et al., *Case Studies in Abdominal and Pelvic Imaging*,
DOI: 10.1007/978-0-85729-366-4_62, © Springer-Verlag London Limited 2011

Answers

1. The US shows a longitudinal view of the right kidney, the adjacent right lobe of the liver (*horizontal arrow* Image 3) and fluid (*long vertical arrow* Image 3) between the right lobe of the liver and the right hemidiaphragm (*short vertical arrows* Image 3).
2. The CXR shows mild elevation of the right hemidiaphragm (*vertical arrow* Image 4) and an air fluid level beneath it (*horizontal arrows* Image 4).
3. A subphrenic collection as a complication of the caesarean section.

The axial and coronal MDCT views in Images 5a and b confirm the subphrenic collection from which frank pus was drained percutaneously. In any septic patient, an elevated hemidiaphragm on a CXR, with or without an air fluid level, should raise the suspicion of a subphrenic collection. This can be quickly confirmed or refuted by US. However, MDCT can clearly delineate the collection.

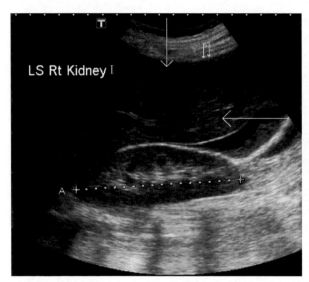

Image 3

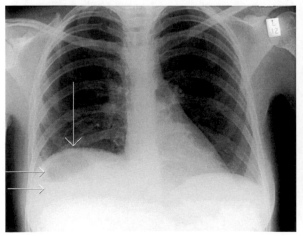

Image 4

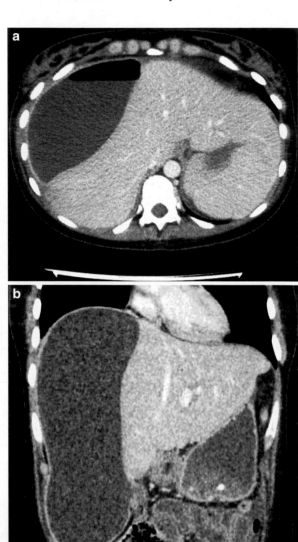

Image 5

Key Points

> Elevated hemidiaphragm in septic patient, consider subphrenic collection.
> US can quickly confirm or refute diagnosis.
> MDCT accurately delineates the collection and is helpful for planning percutaneous drainage.

Further Reading

Geoghegan T and Lee MJ (2007) Emergency radiology, imaging and intervention in sepsis, ISBN 978-3-540-26227-5, 471-480. Springer Berlin Heidelberg

Case 63

A 45-year-old male was reviewed in outpatients. He gave a history of abdominal discomfort and weight loss.

A CT scan is performed.

Questions

1. What are the CT findings?
2. What are the possible diagnoses?

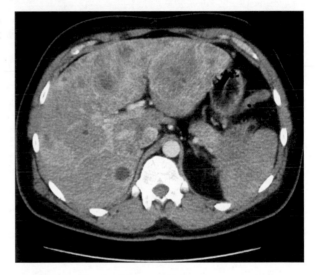

Image 1

R. Joarder et al., *Case Studies in Abdominal and Pelvic Imaging*,
DOI: 10.1007/978-0-85729-366-4_63, © Springer-Verlag London Limited 2011

Answers

1. The scan has been performed in the arterial phase. Note the relatively high attenuation in the aorta compared to a venous phase scan. There are multiple abnormalities within the liver (Image 2 *black arrow*). These are of mixed attenuation and show evidence of increased enhancement, particularly peripherally rim enhancement in comparison with the adjacent liver parenchyma. In addition there is a 4-cm predominately low attenuation abnormality in the tail of the pancreas (*white arrow*). There is stranding of the adjacent peripancreatic fat.
2. The features most in keeping with a pancreatic neoplasm and hepatic metastases.

Alternatively the pancreatic lesion could also be metastatic from another primary.

The hypervascular nature of the liver metastases raises the possibility of a neuroendocrine tumour. A renal cell carcinoma could also account for both hypervascular liver metastases and a pancreatic deposit.

Most hepatic metastases derive their blood supply from the hepatic artery. They are however generally less vascular than surrounding tissue and therefore show relatively reduced attenuation in both arterial and venous phases.

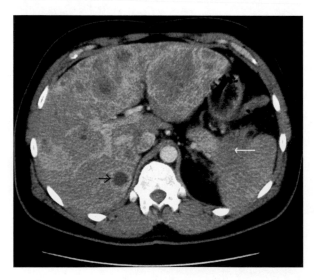

Image 2

Lesions that have increased vascularity compared with normal tissue will show increased enhancement and are termed hypervascular.

Hypervascular liver metastases are found in the following conditions:

Renal cell cancer
Carcinoid
Pancreatic islet cell tumour
Breast cancer
Melanoma
Sarcoma
Neuroendocrine tumours, e.g. phaeochromocytoma

Other hypervascular focal hepatic abnormalities include:

Hepatocellular carcinoma
Focal nodular hyperplasia
Adenoma
Haemangioma

Metastases to the pancreas from other primary sites are uncommon. It is quoted as occurring in 3–10% at autopsy. The commonest primary sites are renal cell lung and breast.

Key Points

> Most hepatic metastases show reduced enhancement in comparison with normal liver parenchyma.
> Hypervascular lesions show increased enhancement and this may act as an aid to diagnosis.
> Metastatic spread of disease to the pancreas is uncommon.

Further Reading

Marin D, Nelson R, Samei E et al (2009) Hypervascular Liver Tumors: Low Tube Voltage, High Tube Current Multidetector CT during Late Hepatic Arterial Phase for Detection—Initial Clinical Experience. Radiology 251 (3) 771-9

A 55-year-old female presented with a 1-year history of seizures, episodic confusion and personality change. At the time of a seizure blood glucose was markedly low.

An MDCT of the abdomen was performed (Images 1 and 2 Axial CT in the arterial phase).

Questions

1. What organ is arrowed?
2. Describe the abnormality in that organ.
3. What is the likely diagnosis?

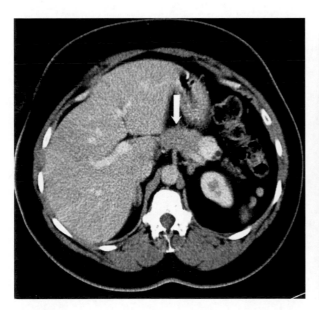

Image 1

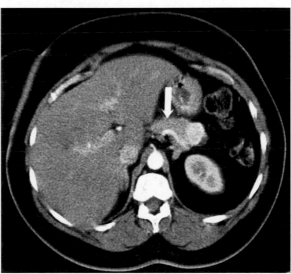

Image 2

R. Joarder et al., *Case Studies in Abdominal and Pelvic Imaging*,
DOI: 10.1007/978-0-85729-366-4_64, © Springer-Verlag London Limited 2011

Answers

1. Pancreas (*long arrows* Images 3 and 4).
2. Avidly enhancing, well-defined mass in the body of the pancreas (*short arrows* Images 3 and 4).
3. Insulinoma.

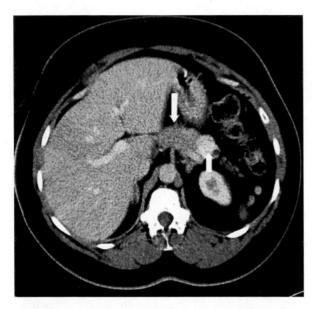

Image 3

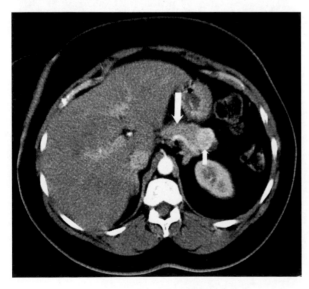

Image 4

Insulinomas are rare neuroendocrine tumours – with an incidence of approximately 4 per million per year. They may be a sporadic or as part of multiple endocrine neoplasia type 1 (MEN1). Insulinomas are usually benign (90%). In sporadic cases they are usually solitary (95%) and in MEN1 they are often multiple (90%).

They usually present with neurogylcopenic or hypoglycaemic symptoms.

The diagnosis should be established biochemically – elevated plasma insulin and C-peptide during biochemical hypoglycaemia (plasma glucose <2.2 mM).

Once the biochemical diagnosis is made it is necessary to locate the tumour. Most are intrapancreatic but they may be ectopic or even occult.

MDCT in both arterial and venous phases may demonstrate an avidly enhancing well-defined tumour in the pancreas which demonstrates rapid washout. MRI, angiography (with stimulation and sampling) and ultrasound (transabdominal, EUS, intraoperative) have all been described as imaging modalities.

Surgical resection, enucleation in solitary tumours and pancreatectomy in multiple tumours is often curative.

Inoperable or metastatic tumours may be treated with other modalities such as chemotherapy, radiofrequency ablation, etc.

Key Points

> Insulinomas often present with symptoms due to hypoglycaemia.
> The diagnosis should be established biochemically.
> MDCT is used to indentify avidly enhancing tumour with rapid contrast washout – usually in the pancreas.

Further Readings

Alexakis N, Neoptolemos JP. (2008) Pancreatic neuroendocrine tumours. Best Pract Res Clin Gastroenterol 22(1): 183-205
Mathur A, Gorden P, Libutti SK. (2009) Insulinoma. Surg Clin North Am 89(5):1105-21

A 74-year-old man presented to his GP with left leg swelling. A Doppler US was performed and the deep veins of the left leg and thigh were patent with no thrombus. An US of the abdomen revealed a solid mass adjacent to the aorta, and therefore a CT was performed (Images 1a and b).

Questions

1. What do Images 1a and b show?
2. How does this explain the patient's symptoms?
3. What is the most likely diagnosis?

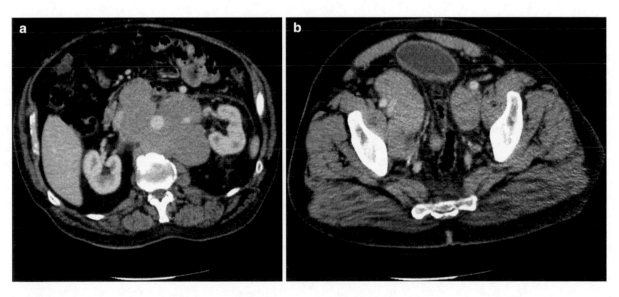

Image 1

Answers

1. The CT shows extensive para-aortic lymphade-nopathy (Image 2a) and bilateral iliac lymphade-nopathy (Image 2b). On the left the left iliac lymphadenopathy is compressing the left common iliac vein.
2. The compression of the left common iliac vein is the cause of the left leg swelling.
3. Lymphoma.

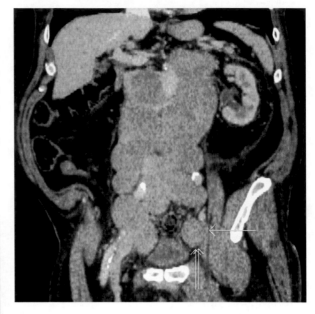

Image 3

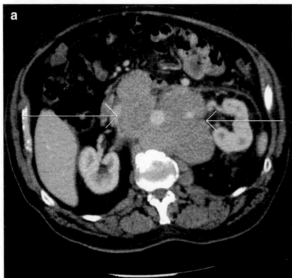

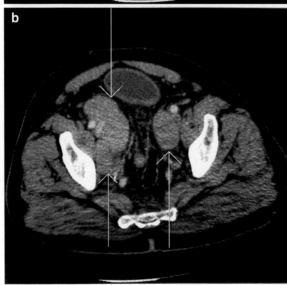

Image 2

CT is the imaging modality of choice to stage, plan biopsies and follow up response to treatment of both Hodgkin's and non-Hodgkin's lymphoma. Every organ can be involved, therefore a systematic examination of a CT of the thorax, abdomen and pelvis is required.

The coronal reconstruction (Image 3) clearly shows the extensive para-aortic and iliac lymphadenopathy. The left iliac nodes (*double arrow*) are compressing the left common iliac vein (*single arrow*).

Key Points

> Leg swelling can be due to a proximal compression of the iliac or femoral veins with or without the presence of a deep vein thrombosis.
> Lymphoma is the most common (but not exclusive) cause of extensive intra-abdominal and pelvic lymphadenopathy.

Further Reading

E.K.Fishman et al (1991) CT of Lymphoma: Spectrum of disease. Radiographics, 11, 647-669

An 85-year-old man was referred for investigation as an out patient. He gave a history of gradually increasing upper abdominal discomfort and pain with some weight loss.

On examination he had hepatomegaly.

MDCT of his abdomen was performed.

Questions

1. What does the CT show?
2. In what percent of cases does malignant degeneration occur?
3. What are the treatment options?

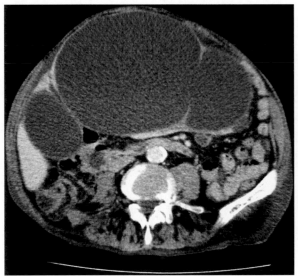

Image 1

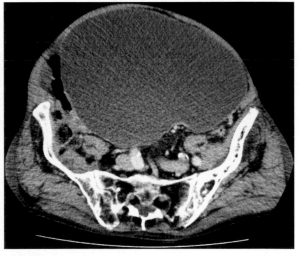

Image 2

R. Joarder et al., *Case Studies in Abdominal and Pelvic Imaging*,
DOI: 10.1007/978-0-85729-366-4_66, © Springer-Verlag London Limited 2011

Answers

1. The CT shows multiple low attenuation areas in the liver. Some are large with a very large region extending inferiorly. The features are those of multiple liver cysts. The extremely large cyst extending inferiorly is the cause of the patient's discomfort.
2. Whilst case reports exist of carcinoma arising in apparently simple liver cysts malignant transformation is extremely rare.
3. Treatment options include radiological and surgical interventions; radiological intervention includes cyst aspiration and sclerosis. Recurrence is frequent. Surgical management includes open or laparoscopic fenestration, liver resection with fenestration.

The majority of liver cysts are sporadic in nature and asymptomatic. Cases of multiple cysts occur in adult polycystic liver disease (PCLD). This is an autosomal dominant (AD) condition that is associated with AD polycystic kidney disease (APCKD), but can occur in isolation. Whilst generally asymptomatic liver enlargement can lead to symptoms of abdominal pain, early satiety, nausea, and dyspnoea.

Complications of PCLD include cyst rupture, torsion haemorrhage and infection. Portal hypertension, biliary obstruction, ascites and peripheral oedema are reported, as is malignancy. There is an association with intracranial aneurysms (as with APCKD) and valvular heart disease.

Treatment is as before with transplantation as an ultimate option.

The diagnosis of a simple liver cyst is usually made on ultrasound. On CT it can be difficult to fully evaluate small cysts. MRI is very useful for differentiating simple cysts from more complex abnormalities. This may be important in patients with an underlying malignancy to differentiate simple cysts (or haemangioma) from metastatic disease.

Sequences included heavily weighted T2 and post-gadolinium. The value of MRI diffusion weighted imaging (DWI) is the subject of investigation.

In this case CT was performed as a first rather than ultrasound as there were concerns regarding underlying malignancy as a cause of the hepatomegaly.

Key Points

> Most hepatic cysts are coincidental asymptomatic findings.
> Radiological drainage is a relatively simple repeatable treatment option for symptomatic cysts.
> Recurrence is common and may be rapid.

Further Reading

Sandrasegaran K, Akisik F, Lin C, Tahir B, Rajan J, Aisen A (2009) The value of diffusion-weighted imaging in characterizing focal liver masses. Acad Radiol. 16(10):1208-14

Case 67

A 57-year-old previously fit male presented with weight loss and back pain. CRP was elevated at 80.

MDCT abdomen was performed (Image 1, axial of mid abdomen; and Image 2, coronal MPR both in arterial phase).

Questions

1. What abnormality is demonstrated?
2. What are the possible causes?

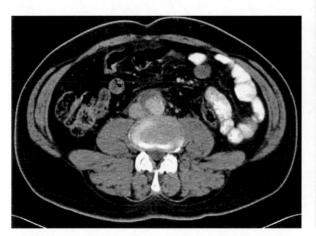

Image 1

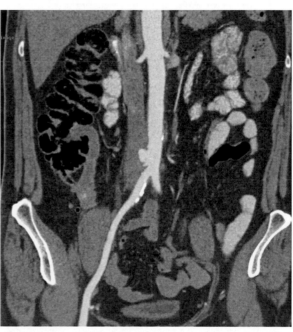

Image 2

R. Joarder et al., *Case Studies in Abdominal and Pelvic Imaging*,
DOI: 10.1007/978-0-85729-366-4_67, © Springer-Verlag London Limited 2011

Answers

1. There is a 2-cm eccentric aneurysm arising from the right side of the lower aorta compressing the IVC (*arrows* Images 3 and 4).
2. Saccular aneurysm of the lower abdominal aorta – causes include atherosclerosis, penetrating aortic ulcer, trauma (unusual at this site) or infection (mycotic).

Blood cultures were negative but the CT and clinical presentation suggested a mycotic cause. Intravenous antibiotics were commenced.

Traditionally mycotic aneurysms have been treated surgically – aneurysm excision, aortic grafting or even aortic excision with extra-anatomic bypass.

However as an alternative to difficult and dangerous surgery it was decided to treat the aneurysm with endovascular aneurysm repair (EVAR) (Image 5 *arrows* on stent graft being deployed over mycotic aneurysm). A covered aorto-uni-iliac stent graft was placed across the aneurysm and a femoro-femoro graft placed to supply the left leg. The patient was placed on lifelong oral antibiotics.

The patient was asymptomatic during follow-up and the CT at 2 years shows resolution of the aneurysm with no complications of EVAR (Image 6 *arrows* on stent graft).

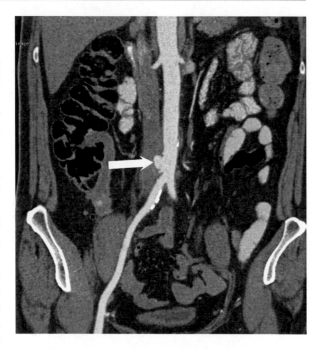

Image 4

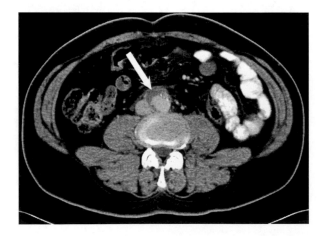

Image 3

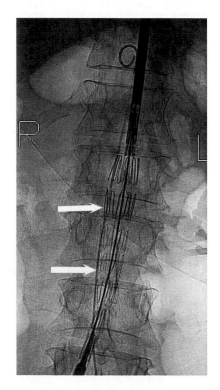

Image 5

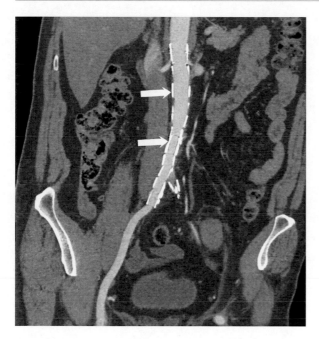

Image 6

> Mycotic aortic aneurysms are rare and often present non-specifically.
> EVAR is replacing conventional surgery as the treatment of choice.

Case 68

A 51-year-old female presented with a 1-month history of increasing abdominal swelling and pain. An MDCT of the abdomen and pelvis were performed (Images 1a–d).

Questions

1. What does Image 1a show?
2. What do Images 1b and c show?
3. What does Image 1d show?
4. What is the most likely diagnosis?

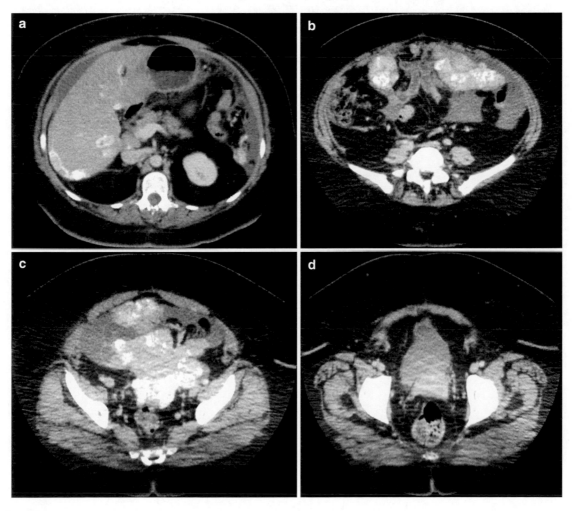

Image 1

R. Joarder et al., *Case Studies in Abdominal and Pelvic Imaging*,
DOI: 10.1007/978-0-85729-366-4_68, © Springer-Verlag London Limited 2011

Answers

1. Ascites (*horizontal arrows* Image 2a) and calcified subcapsular hepatic soft tissue lesions (*vertical arrows* Image 2a).
2. Calcified omental deposits 'omental caking' (Image 2b) and more inferiorly more central lesions (Image 2c).
3. A normal pelvis with no evidence of an ovarian mass.
4. Primary peritoneal carcinoma.

The patient subsequently underwent a biopsy of the omental soft tissue and the diagnosis of primary peritoneal serous carcinoma was made. This condition occurs almost exclusively in women. The usual presentation, as in this case, is of abdominal distension and pain. It is an epithelial tumour that arises from the peritoneum and histopathologically is indistinguishable from metastatic serous ovarian carcinoma. The imaging features are of ascites, peritoneal and omental soft tissue; however, it is the absence of ovarian masses that make the diagnosis more likely than metastatic ovarian carcinoma. The peritoneal nodules can calcify, as in this case.

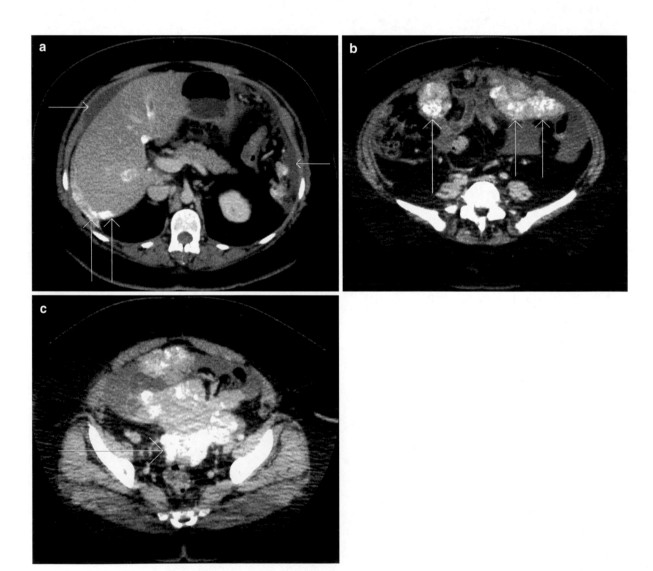

Image 2

Key Point

> Consider primary peritoneal serous carcinoma in presence of peritoneal deposits and ascites in the absence of ovarian masses.

Further Reading

Levy AD et al (2008) Primary peritoneal tumours: Imaging features with pathologic correlation. Radiographics 28,583-607

A 73-year-old woman was seen in the out patients with a history of recurrence of dysphagia. She had been diagnosed with squamous cell carcinoma of the oesophagus 6 months previously and had endoscopic stenting of the distal oesophagus.

Questions

1. What does the CT show?
2. What is the further management?

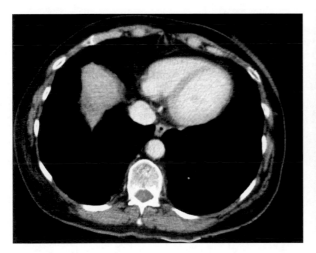

Image 1

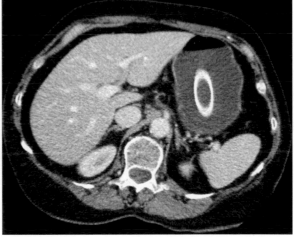

Image 2

R. Joarder et al., *Case Studies in Abdominal and Pelvic Imaging*, DOI: 10.1007/978-0-85729-366-4_69, © Springer-Verlag London Limited 2011

Answers

1. The CT shows thickening of the oesophagus with no evidence of the stent in the oesophagus. There is ovoid high attenuation within the stomach representing the migrated stent (Image 3).
2. A replacement stent could be inserted and the migrated stent recovered.

Endoscopic oesophageal stent insertion is commonly used for the palliation of dysphagia in malignant conditions. It allows for relief of symptoms and enables patients to maintain oral nutrition. A significant improvement in symptoms is seen in the vast majority of patients.

Complications include stent overgrowth, and covered stents are preferred to reduce this. Covered stents are however more likely to migrate, particular those placed in the distal oesophagus or gastro-oesophageal region. Migration rates of 28% are quoted for covered stents.

Stent migration causes recurrence of symptoms. Generally no further harm befalls the patient, although bowel obstruction or perforation are very rare complications. The frequency seems to be increased in patients who have had previous abdominal surgery.

Rarely stents may cause an inflammatory reaction which can lead to a further benign stricture of the oesophagus. Uncovered metal stents may be useful in these circumstance, although are not generally recommended for use in benign conditions.

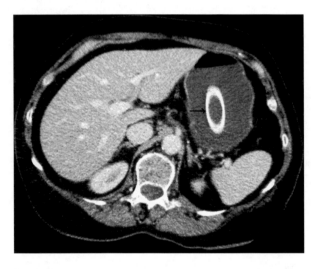

Image 3

Key Points

> Endoscopic stent insertion is useful in palliation of dysphagia in oesophageal cancer.
> Complications include overgrowth and migration.
> Stent migration may be visible on a CXR and should be considered if symptoms recur.

Further Readings

Christie et al Results of expandable metal stents for malignant oesophageal obstruction in 100 patients short-term and long-term follow-up. Ann Thor Surg 71 (6) 1797

M J Metcalfe, A C Steger, and A Leslie. (2004) Benign complications of expandable metal stents used in the palliation of oesophageal carcinoma: two case reports. British Journal of Radiology 77, 245-247

A 30-year-old male known to have sickle cell trait and thalassaemia was investigated for abnormal LFTs and right upper quadrant pain.

MRCP was performed (Image 1, axial T2 weighted image; and Image 2, axial T1 weight image of the liver and spleen).

Questions

1. Describe the signal intensity of both liver and spleen.
2. Comment on the marrow signal in the vertebra.
3. Comment on the spleen.

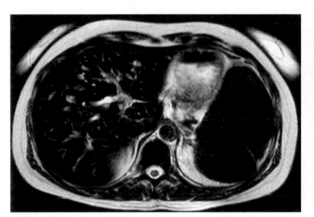

Image 1

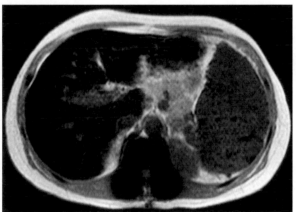

Image 2

R. Joarder et al., *Case Studies in Abdominal and Pelvic Imaging*,
DOI: 10.1007/978-0-85729-366-4_70, © Springer-Verlag London Limited 2011

Answers

1. Both liver (*long arrows* Images 3 and 4) and spleen (*short arrows* Images 3 and 4) show markedly low signal intensity.
2. The marrow signal is also low (*arrowhead* Image 4) (with blooming/chemical shift artefact on the T1 – *stars*).
3. The spleen is enlarged and inhomogeneous.

The findings are due to iron overload from multiple previous blood transfusions for sickle cell trait and thalassaemia.

Classically, serum ferritin and liver biopsy have been used to assess patients and monitor response to chelation therapy.

Recently, MRI has proven effective in detecting and quantifying iron in the heart and liver. Tissue iron is paramagnetic and increases the MRI relaxation rates R2 and R2* in a quantifiable manner [1].

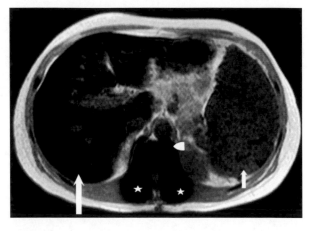

Image 4

The paramagnetic effect of iron decreases the signal intensity on both TI and T2 weighted images giving a dramatic appearance of black liver, spleen and bones.

Key Points

> Iron overload causes low signal in liver, spleen and bone marrow on both T1 and T2 MRI images.
> MRI can be used to quantify iron overload.

Reference

1. Voskaridou E, Douskou M, Terpos E, et al. (2004) Magnetic resonance imaging in the evaluation of iron overload in patients with beta thalasaemia and sickle cell disease. Br J Haematol 126(5):736-42

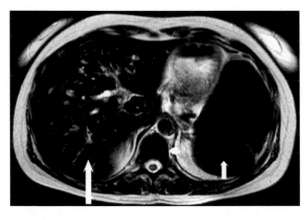

Image 3

Case 71

An 83-year-old female with a long history of urinary incontinence and a permanent urinary catheter presented acutely feeling generally unwell with a blocked catheter and a urinary tract infection. She had type 2 diabetes; past history included hypertension, atrial fibrillation and hysterectomy. On examination she was found to have significant abdominal swelling. She had noticed the swelling increasing over the last three months. On admission the catheter was changed and drained a litre of cloudy urine. An abdominal X-ray (Image 1) was then performed.

Bloods showed a high WBC and urine examination confirmed a high leukocyte count. Other positive findings included normocytic anaemia with haemoglobin of 8.3 g/dL, a Ca 12-5 level was found to be 250 ku/L.

Questions

1. What does Image 1 show?
2. Given the above results, what is the most likely diagnosis?

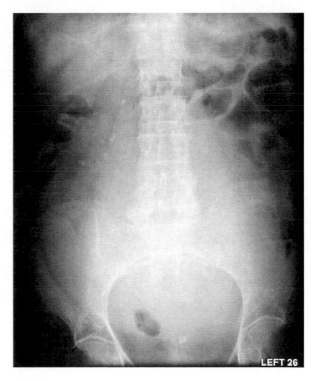

Image 1

Answers

1. The abdominal X-ray showed a well-defined, large mass arising from the pelvis, filling the pelvis and central abdomen displacing bowel loops around it (Image 2).
2. As the bladder had been successfully recatheterised, the appearances are suggestive of a large ovarian cyst (ovaries were preserved at hysterectomy) and given the raised Ca 12-5 it is likely to be malignant.

Having found a significant abdominal mass on examination, ultrasound would be the imaging modality of choice. However, given AXR available, it is important to correctly pick up the abnormality. In addition to evaluating the calibre of large and small bowel loops, it is helpful to note their position and any paucity of bowel gas markings centrally. In this case due to the significant displacement of bowel by the large pelvic mass.

CT confirmed a complex ovarian cyst with soft tissue nodularity at the right lateral and inferior aspect (Images 3a and b). The RMI (risk of malignancy index) [1] is usually calculated using ultrasound rather than CT appearances, the combination of complex cyst with a raised CA-125 in a post-menopausal woman is highly suggestive of an ovarian carcinoma.

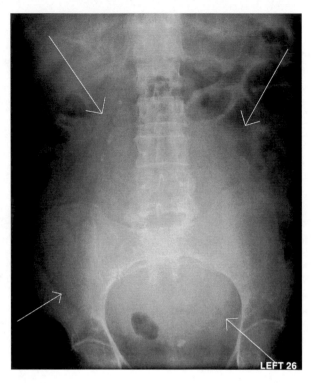

Image 2

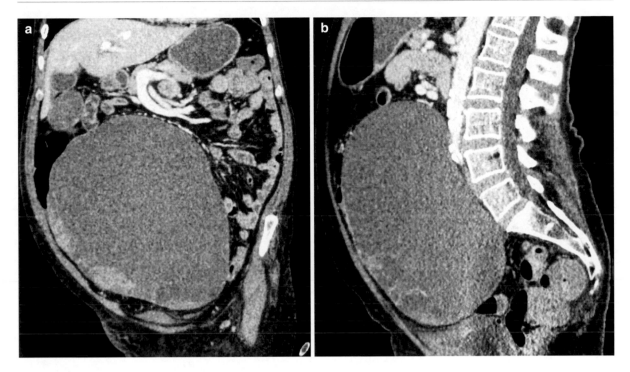

Image 3

Reference

1. T A. Bali and K. Reynolds (2004) The current management of primary ovarian cancer: a review. Cancer Therapy Vol. 2, 305-316

A 66-year-old man underwent investigation for prostate cancer. His PSA was 17. Prostate biopsy confirmed adenocarcinoma with a Gleeson grade greater than 4 + 3.

Isotope bone scan and MRI of the prostate were performed. The isotope bone scan showed no evidence of bone metastases.

Questions

1. What are the image findings?
2. What stage disease does this represent?
3. How does staging affect management?

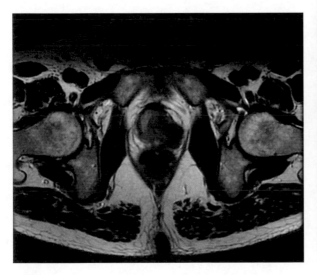

Image 1

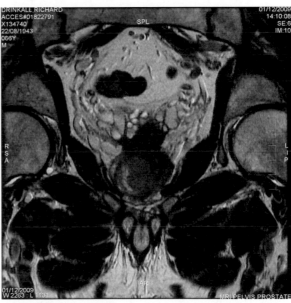

Image 2

R. Joarder et al., *Case Studies in Abdominal and Pelvic Imaging*,
DOI: 10.1007/978-0-85729-366-4_72, © Springer-Verlag London Limited 2011

Answers

1. Image 1 is from an axial T2 weighted series, Image 2 from a coronal T2 weighted series. There is low signal abnormality in the left peripheral zone (Image 3 *white arrow*) that extends beyond the margin of the gland. The *black arrow* on Image 3 indicates the normal gland margin on the right. There is low signal abnormality within the left seminal vesicle (Image 4 *arrow*). There is therefore evidence of extra-capsular spread and disease spread into the adjacent seminal vesicle.
2. The MRI staging is of T3b disease.
3. The treatment options are influenced by staging particularly the presence or absence of localised (organ confined) disease.

Treatment options for prostate cancer are dependant upon staging. Whilst there is a little national variation within patient groups, in general the following applies.

i. For localised disease in patients with a 10–15 year estimated life expectancy, they may be offered a choice of active surveillance, radical surgery (laparoscopic or open) or radiotherapy options (external

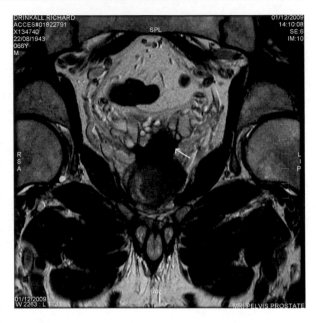

Image 4

beam or brachytherapy) depending upon stage, PSA and Gleeson score.

Surgery would only be considered in exceptional circumstances for patients with less than 10–15 year life expectancy.

ii. Patients in whom disease is locally advanced may be offered hormone manipulation and/or radiotherapy or involvement in a trial.
iii. Patients with metastatic disease may be offered hormone manipulation and/or trial entry.

On T1-weighted images, the prostate demonstrates homogeneous intermediate signal intensity, and tumours are impossible to discern. On T2-weighted images, cancer most commonly demonstrates decreased signal intensity relative to the high-signal intensity normal peripheral zone. Visualisation of disease within the transitional zone is more difficult, although improved by use of endorectal coils, higher field strengths and complimentary techniques.

Post-biopsy haemorrhage may also appear as low signal, and a suitable time interval must be left between biopsy and scanning.

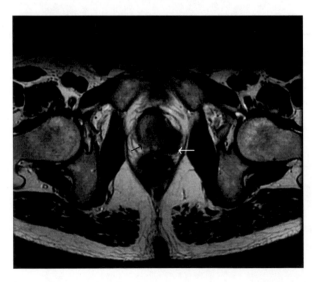

Image 3

Key Points

> Treatment options for prostate cancer depend upon disease stage. Imaging investigation is guided by Gleeson score and PSA.

> Local disease staging is with MRI, the extent of distant bone disease is assessed with radionuclide imaging (bone scan).

Further Reading

Guidance from local cancer networks is published online for example http://www.sussexcancer.net/professionals/clinicalgroups/tumourgroups/urology/

Hricak H, Choyke P, Eberhardt S, Leibel S, Scardino P (2007) Imaging Prostate Cancer: A Multidisciplinary Perspective. Radiology 243 (1) 28-53

A 45-year-old male inpatient, being treated for alcohol-induced chronic pancreatitis, complained of sudden-onset severe abdominal pain associated with tachycardia and falling haemoglobin. The patient was presumed to be bleeding into the abdomen and a contrast-enhanced MDCT was performed (Images 1 and 2 Axial, non-contiguous, CTs of the upper abdomen).

Questions

1. Comment on the appearance of the pancreas.
2. What are the rounded enhancing serpiginous structures adjacent of the pancreatic head?
3. What is the large mixed attenuation mass just below the pancreas?

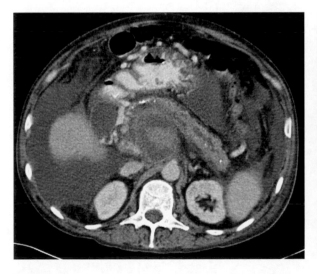

Image 1

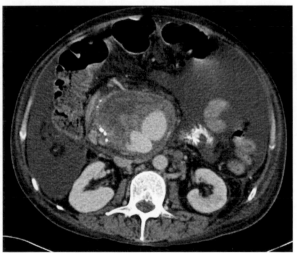

Image 2

R. Joarder et al., *Case Studies in Abdominal and Pelvic Imaging*, DOI: 10.1007/978-0-85729-366-4_73, © Springer-Verlag London Limited 2011

Answers

1. There is pancreatic calcification (*medium arrow* Image 3) and pancreatic duct dilatation (*short arrow* Image 3) consistent with chronic pancreatitis.
2. These are dilated peribiliary veins (*long arrow* Image 3) – cavernous transformation – secondary to portal vein thrombosis due to chronic pancreatitis.
3. This is a large ruptured false aneurysm (*short arrow* on "lumen" of false aneurysm and *long arrow* on surrounding haematoma Image 4) secondary to chronic pancreatitis.

Chronic pancreatitis has many complications. This case illustrates a vascular complication. It is thought that chronic inflammation and pancreatic secretions cause local arteritis and weakening of the arterial wall and thus false aneurysm formation. These false aneurysms are at risk of rupture and therefore life threatening haemorrhage. Any peripancreatic artery can be affected, most commonly the gastroduodenal or splenic arteries.

This case was treated endovascularly. Angiography demonstrated the aneurysm arising from the superior mesenteric artery (*arrows* Image 5). It was not possible to coil the aneurysm due to its wide neck and large size. As the patient was exsanguinating and not fit for surgery endovascular control of haemorrhage was vital and therefore thrombin was injected through the catheter into the false aneurysm. This caused the aneurysm to thrombose and the haemorrhage to stop immediately (Image 6) and not recur. There was a small amount of thrombin-induced clot distally in the SMA, but this was asymptomatic, did not cause bowel ischaemia and was not present on follow-up MDCT.

A better treatment option would have been a covered stent graft in the SMA across the false aneurysm neck, but this was not available.

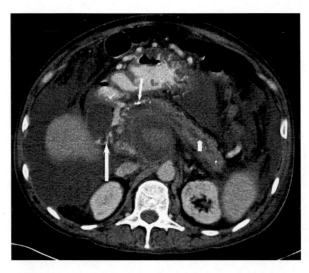

Image 3

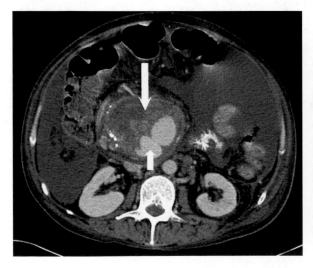

Image 4

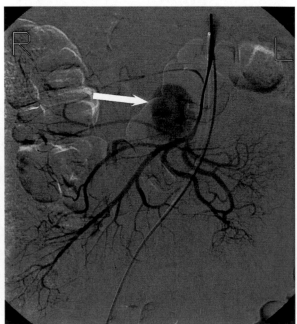

Image 5

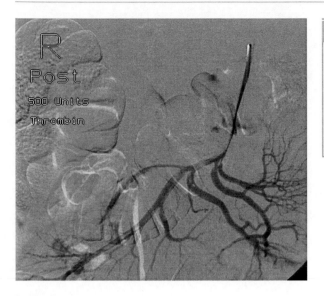

Image 6

> False aneurysms are a well-recognised vascular complication of chronic pancreatitis.
> Endovascular techniques – embolisation or stent grafting is the preferred method of preventing and treating rupture.

An 87-year-old male presented with a 5-week history of pneumaturia and recurrent urinary tract infection. An MDCT of the abdomen and pelvis was performed (Images 1a–c).

Questions

1. What does Image 1a show?
2. What does Images 1b show?
3. What does Image 1c show?
4. What is the diagnosis?

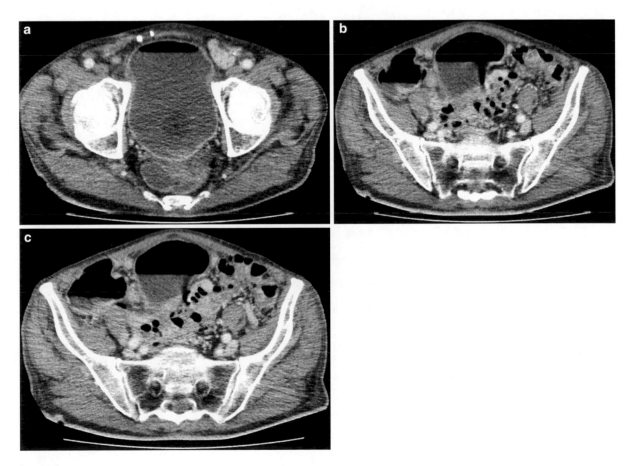

Image 1

Answers

1. An air fluid level within the bladder.
2. A jet of air within the left side of the bladder extending from posterior to anterior to join the air already present (Image 2a).
3. A diverticulum which is continuous with the air jet (Image 2b).
4. A colovesical fistula as a complication of diverticular disease.

The sagittal reconstruction (Image 3) delineates the fistula clearly with the air jet just caught at the time of scanning. The symptoms of recurrent urinary tract infection and pneumaturia are pathognomonic for colovesical fistula. The most common cause is diverticular disease. If CT is performed to confirm the diagnosis, it can be helpful to instil dilute (2% strength)

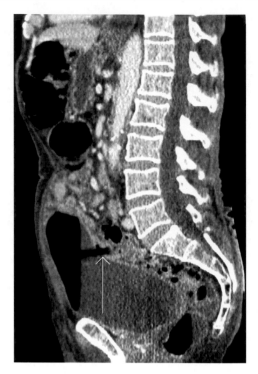

Image 3

positive contrast per rectum prior to scanning. If contrast is seen within the bladder, there must be a connection between it and the colon. However, as in this case, the tract may be identified continuous with a diverticulum without positive rectal contrast.

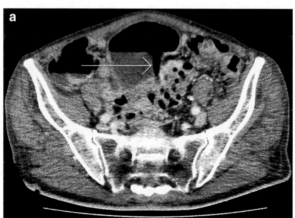

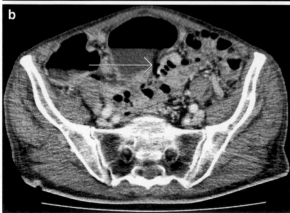

Image 2

Key Points

> Diverticular disease is the most common cause of colovesical fistula.
> The presence of air within an uncatheterised bladder is highly suggestive of the diagnosis.
> Positive rectal contrast prior to CT scanning can increase the detection of fistula.

Further Reading

Melchior S et al (2009) Diagnosis and surgical management of colovesical fistulas due to sigmid diverticulitis. J Urol 182 (3) 978-82

An 80-year-old female was undergoing investigation for microscopic heamaturia. Flexible cystoscopy is normal. A CT urogram (CTU) is performed.

Questions

1. What do Images 1 and 2 show?
2. What does Image 3 show?
3. How would you stage this abnormality?
4. What are the treatment options?

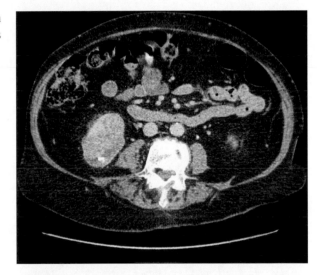

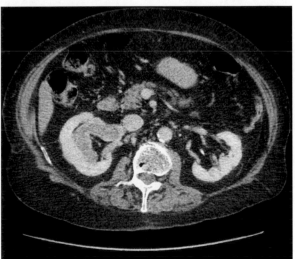

Image 2

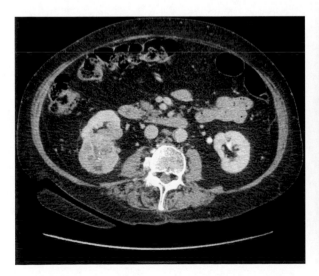

Image 1

Image 3

R. Joarder et al., *Case Studies in Abdominal and Pelvic Imaging*,
DOI: 10.1007/978-0-85729-366-4_75, © Springer-Verlag London Limited 2011

Answers

1. There is a mixed attenuation region replacing the posterior mid portion and lower pole of the right kidney (Image 4). This contains low attenuation and calcific density. The features are those of a renal neoplasm, most likely a renal cell carcinoma.
2. There is a relative low attenuation curvilinear region within the hilum of the right kidney extending towards the IVC (Image 5). This represents an expanded renal vein containing tumour thrombus.
3. Staging of renal cancers is as follows:

   T1 tumour confined to kidney and less than 7 cm

   T2 tumour confined to kidney and greater than 7 cm

   T3a tumour invades adrenal gland or perinephric tissues but not beyond Gerota fascia

   T3b extension into renal vein or IVC below diaphragm

   T3c extension into IVC above diaphragm

   T4 tumour invades below Gerota fascia

   N0 no regional lymph node disease

   N2 single regional lymph node involved

   N2 more than one regional lymph node involved

   In this case staging would be T3b N0.

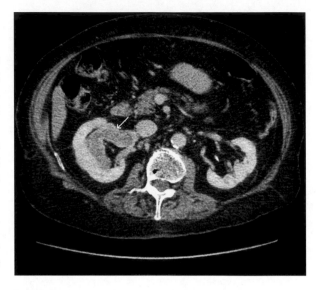

Image 5

4. Treatment options have expanded from traditional open nephrectomy. Laparoscopic surgery in increasing and laparoscopic partial nephrectomy is the probable treatment of choice for tumours under 4 cm (T1a)

Other less-invasive operative and percutaneous techniques include cryotherapy and radiofrequency ablation.

Key Points

> Renal tumours are often found incidentally and are often large at presentation.
> Renal vein extension alters staging and treatment options.

Further Reading

Pouliot F, Shuch B, Larochelle J (2010) Contemporary Management of Renal Tumors With Venous Tumor Thrombus. J Urol Jul 17 epub

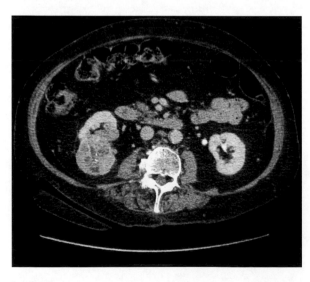

Image 4

A 55-year-old female who had previously received a renal transplant presented with intermittent central abdominal pain. An MDCT of the abdomen was performed with oral and intravenous contrast (Image 1 axial of upper abdomen). Comparison with a previous MDCT performed for haematuria some months earlier was made (Image 2 axial of upper abdomen).

Questions

1. Why did the patient require a renal transplant?
2. Comment on the pancreas.
3. Is there any other abnormality visible?
4. What had changed compared to the previous CT?

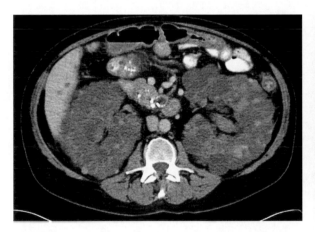

Image 1

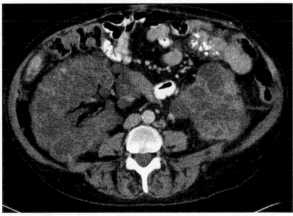

Image 2

R. Joarder et al., *Case Studies in Abdominal and Pelvic Imaging*,
DOI: 10.1007/978-0-85729-366-4_76, © Springer-Verlag London Limited 2011

Answers

1. She had adult polycystic kidney disease (*long arrows* Image 3).
2. The pancreas contains calcification (*short arrow* Image 3).
3. The is a mass anterior to the pancreas – similar in appearance to the pancreas and also containing calcification (*medium arrows* Image 3).
4. The mass had moved from the left upper quadrant (*arrow* Image 4) to anterior to the pancreas (*medium arrow* Image 3).

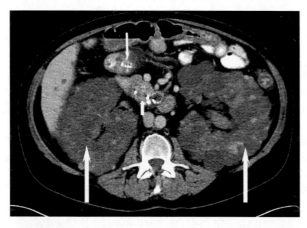

Image 3

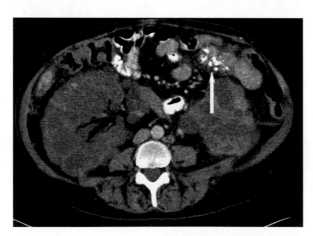

Image 4

The mass was thought to be the cause of the abdominal pain and it was removed laparoscopically. The abdominal pain resolved and histological analysis of the specimen revealed 'chronic pancreatitis of heterotopic pancreas'.

Heterotopic pancreas is a congenital anomaly where aberrant pancreas is without ductal or vascular continuity with the gland. It is often discovered incidentally during imaging and true incidence is unknown, but estimates vary from 1% to 14%. The most common site of the ectopic pancreatic tissue is the upper GI tract. In the case presented above the ectopic tissue was located in the wall of the proximal jejunum – accounting for its mobility. Heterotopic pancreas can be subject to all same disease processes as the native gland including pancreatitis and adenocarcinoma. In this case both the native and ectopic pancreatic tissue show signs of chronic pancreatitis, and on closer questioning there was a history of previous alcohol misuse.

Symptoms are varied but include epigastric pain, weight loss, bleeding and bowel obstruction. Imaging is often non-specific, but occasionally a dilated duct can be seen running through the tissue. Diagnosis is therefore often made at biopsy or surgery.

Key Points

> Heterotopic pancreas is probably fairly common.
> It presents non-specifically both clinically and radiologically.
> Diagnosis is often only made at biopsy or removal.
> The heterotopic pancreas can undergo the same disease processes as the native gland.

Further Reading

Kung JW, Brown A, Kruskal JB et al (2010) Heterotopic pancreas: typical and atypical imaging findings. Clin Radiol 65:403-407

A 60-year-old female presented with a 5-week history of rectal bleeding and occasional loose stools but no other persistent change in bowel habit. An MRI (sagittal, axial and coronal T2 scans) was performed through the rectum (Images 1a–c).

Questions

1. What do Images 1a–c show?
2. What is the diagnosis?
3. Is the abnormality operable with curative intent if there is no disease elsewhere?
4. What treatment is most likely to be offered?

R. Joarder et al., *Case Studies in Abdominal and Pelvic Imaging*,
DOI: 10.1007/978-0-85729-366-4_77, © Springer-Verlag London Limited 2011

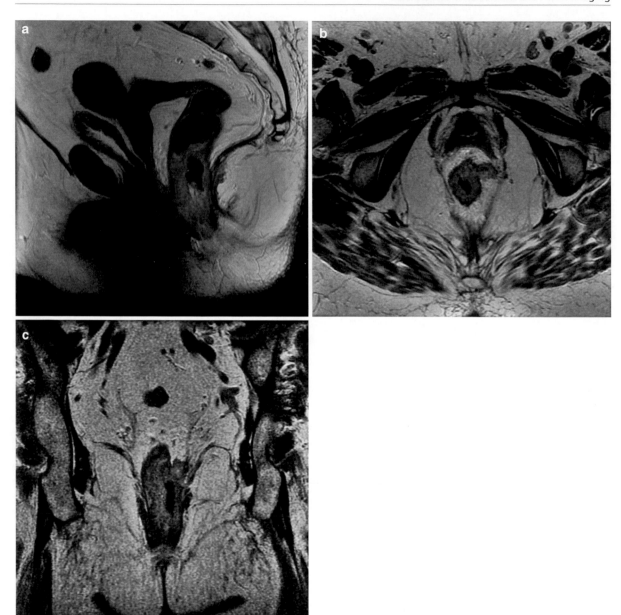

Image 1

Answers

1. The MRI shows abnormal soft tissue within the rectum commencing approximately 1 cm above the dentate line, extending anteriorly to involve the posterior vaginal wall, laterally to involve the left lateral mesorectal fascia and inferiolaterally to involve the left levator muscle. No lymphadenopathy was identified.

2. A locally extensive low rectal tumour.

3. The involvement of the vagina (Image 2a), the mesorectal fascia (Image 2b) and left levator (Image 2c) makes this low rectal tumour inoperable without downstaging.

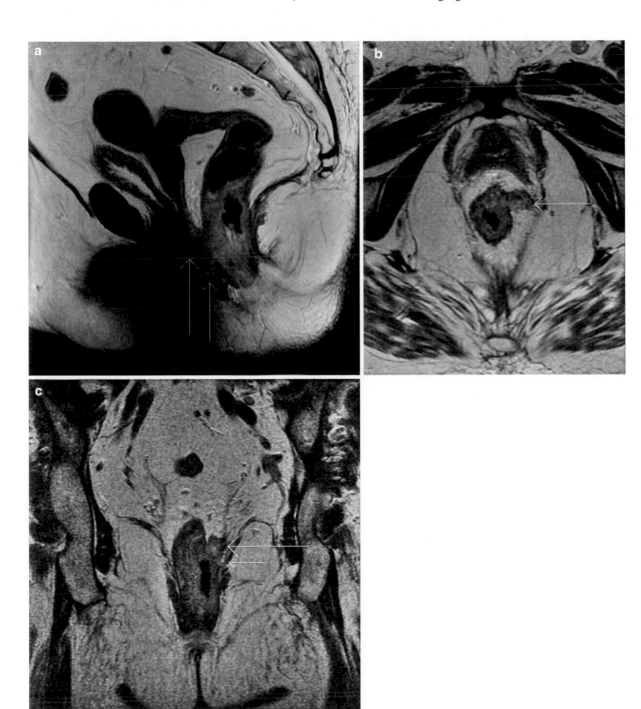

Image 2

4. The patient may be offered long-course chemo-radiotherapy to downstage the tumour to 'operable' prior to an abdominoperineal excision.

Accurate staging of rectal tumours is essential to minimise involvement of the surgical resection margin. This is particularly important for low rectal tumours treated by abdominoperineal resection as they have a higher rate of margin involvement than tumours higher up in the rectum. Careful imaging assessment with MRI allows the radiologist to demonstrate whether the surgical planes are tumour free or involved. The resection margin is said to be 'threatened' when tumour is within 1 mm of the mesorectal fascia. If this is the case, a decision can then be made regarding downstaging chemo-radiotherapy prior to curative surgery or whether the patient follows a palliative treatment pathway.

Clearly, CT staging of the chest and upper abdomen is required to identify distant metastases.

The important areas to review are:

1. Tumour height (from dentate line).
2. Tumour position relating to anterior peritoneal reflection (not seen on the images given above).
3. T staging of tumour, is it breaching the wall of the rectum (T3) and if so by how much?
4. How far from the mesorectal fascia (MSF) is the tumour? If 1 mm or greater from the MRF (Image 3)?
5. Is there nodal involvement and if so is an involved node within 1 mm of the MRF?
6. Are the levator muscles involved?
7. Is there involvement of adjacent organs, e.g. vagina/bladder/prostate?
8. Is there pelvic side wall lymphadenopathy?

Key Points

> ❯ Careful local staging with MRI is required for all potentially operable rectal tumours.
> ❯ Low rectal cancers have a higher rate of margin involvement than higher rectal tumours.

Further Reading

Shihab OC et al (2009) MRI staging of low rectal cancer.; European Radiology 19(3) 643-650

A 30-year-old woman is seen in the Emergency Department with a history of increasing flank pain. She is 4 months post-partum. Urinalysis reveals dipstick haematuria.

MDCT of the abdomen and pelvis is performed.

Questions

1. What are the CT findings?
2. What is the diagnosis?
3. What are the predisposing factors and what is the treatment?

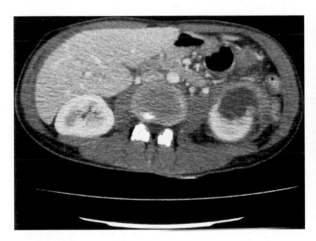

Image 1

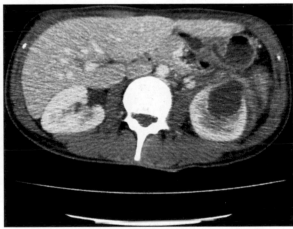

Image 2

R. Joarder et al., *Case Studies in Abdominal and Pelvic Imaging*,
DOI: 10.1007/978-0-85729-366-4_78, © Springer-Verlag London Limited 2011

Answers

1. The CT shows a hypo-attenuating focal region in the lower pole of the left kidney (Image 3 *long arrow*). The wall is thick and irregular. There is alteration of attenuation in the perinephric fat (*short arrow*). There is no dilatation of the collecting system.
2. The features are those of a renal abscess. The perinephric stranding raises the possibility of perinephric spread but may simply represent inflammation rather than contiguous spread of infected material. The only differential diagnosis of concern is a cystic renal carcinoma.
3. Diabetes is a strong predisposing factor. Treatment, in the absence of renal obstruction, is with antibiotics.

A renal abscess may arise as a result of ascending infection or haematogenous spread. The former is more common (4:1). Ascending infection is usually associated with obstruction of the collecting system. Haematogenous spread reflects infection elsewhere but also occurs in IV drug users.

Urinalysis and culture may be negative for cells or blood in up to 20% of cases. This reflects a lesion located purely within the parenchyma.

A cystic renal carcinoma could have similar appearances. Presentation would usually be different unless the primary abnormality acted as a focus of infection. Serial imaging post-abscess treatment is required to ensure resolution of the abnormality which can often be done with US.

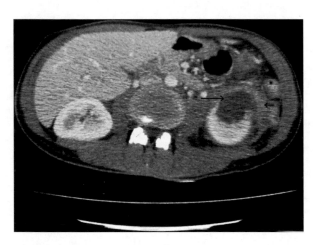

Image 3

Key Points

> Renal abscess is usually a result of ascending infection, and obstructions need to be excluded.
> US follow up is required to ensure resolution.

Further Reading

Dembry LM, Andriole VT. (1997) Renal and perirenal abscesses. Infect Dis Clin North Am 11(3):663-80

A 74-year-old male who had previously suffered from diverticulitis presented with acute lower abdominal pain. A presumptive diagnosis of diverticulitis was made and treatment with intravenous antibiotics commenced. However, the lower abdominal pain worsened and localised diverticular perforation was suspected.

MDCT of the abdomen and pelvis (portal venous phase) was performed (Image 1 – Axial, Image 2 – Coronal).

Questions

1. What is the structure arrowed on the two images?
2. Describe its pattern of enhancement?
3. What is the diagnosis?

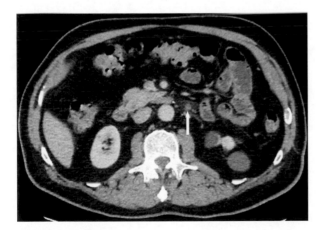

Image 1

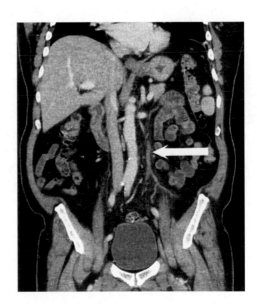

Image 2

R. Joarder et al., *Case Studies in Abdominal and Pelvic Imaging*,
DOI: 10.1007/978-0-85729-366-4_79, © Springer-Verlag London Limited 2011

Answers

1. Inferior mesenteric vein (*arrows* on Images 3 and 4).
2. It is not enhancing.
3. Acute inferior mesenteric vein thrombosis secondary to diverticulitis.

Thrombosis of the inferior mesenteric vein (IMV) is uncommon and usually secondary to diverticulitis or colon cancer. Although the presentation is non-specific, and also depends on the underlying cause, the CT appearances are characteristic – the IMV is distended, ill-defined, non-enhancing or contains filling defect. Treating the underlying cause and anticoagulation (to stop proximal clot propagation) is usually advised.

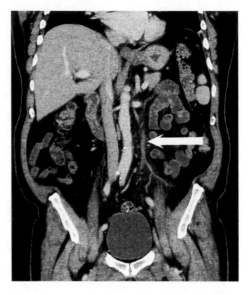

Image 4

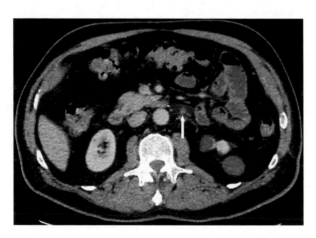

Image 3

Key Points

> IMV thrombosis presents non-specifically.
> Contrast-enhanced CT is usually diagnostic.

Further Reading

Akpinar E, Turkbey B, Karcaaltincaba M, et al. (2008) MDCT of inferior mesenteric vein: normal anatomy and pathology. Clin Radiol 63(7):819-23

A 42-year-old female presented with acute abdominal pain. On examination there was a palpable mass in the RUQ. An AXR (Image 1) and CT of the abdomen and pelvis (Image 2) were performed.

Questions

1. What does Image 1 show?
2. What does Image 2 show?
3. What is the diagnosis?
4. What are the names of the sign seen in Images 1 and 2?

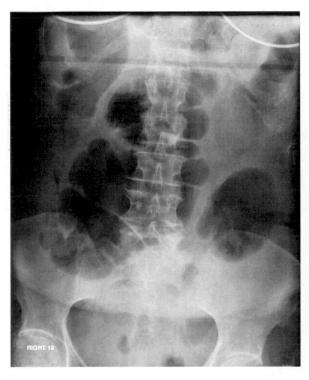

Image 1

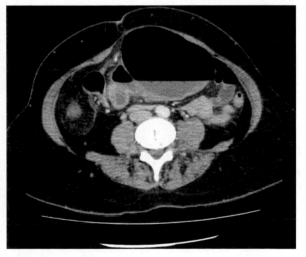

Image 2

R. Joarder et al., *Case Studies in Abdominal and Pelvic Imaging*,
DOI: 10.1007/978-0-85729-366-4_80, © Springer-Verlag London Limited 2011

Answers

1. The AXR shows a large dilated loop of bowel (Image 3) and the rest of the large bowel is undilated.
2. The CT appearance of the AXR showing a grossly dilated caecum seen centrally within the epigastrium, a tapered twisted colon just proximal to the caecum with adjacent swirling of vessels (*oblique arrow* Image 4) and an undistended descending colon (*vertical arrow* Image 4).
3. A caecal volvulus.
4. The "coffee bean sign" on the plain abdominal X-ray and the 'parrot beak' or 'bird of prey' sign (See below).

Caecal volvulus is less common than sigmoid volvulus (11% of intestinal volvulus) in patients ranging from 30 to 60 years old. When the appearances are as in Image 1 the plain film is diagnostic and urgent surgical referral is warranted; however if the caecum is fluid filled the appearances may be atypical. The so-called coffee bean sign refers to the shape of the distended

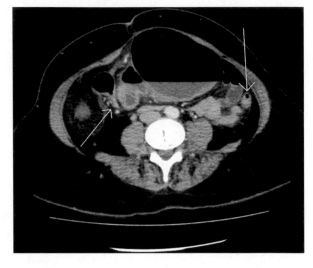

Image 4

caecal pole and is different from the coffee bean sign in sigmoid volvulus which is due to the central opaque line caused by opposing distended loops of sigmoid up against the mesentery on a supine film. Likewise, the 'bird of prey' or 'parrot beak' sign is also seen in sigmoid volvulus both on CT and contrast enema, whereas in cases of caecal volvulus we see the sign on CT only (Image 4 *oblique arrow*). It is due to the tapering bowel at the site of the twist.

Key Points

> Plain AXR may be diagnostic.
> If AXR is not diagnostic or wish to assess for associated malignancy CT can be helpful.
> Look for coffee bean sign on plain AXR.
> Look for bird of prey sign on CT.
> Refer to surgeons urgently if significant dilatation, do not delay by requesting further imaging.

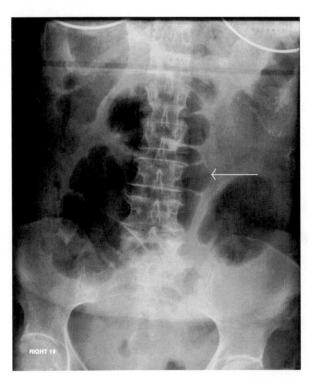

Image 3

Further Reading

Carolyn J Moore et al (2001) CT of Cecal Volvulus. American Journal of Roentgenology 177:95-98

A 61-year-old with a history of invasive ductal carcinoma of the breast has a CT for follow-up of lung nodules.

An abnormality related to the right kidney is seen.

Questions

1. What is the abnormality?
2. What is the Bosniak classification and how would you classify this abnormality?
3. What is the management of this abnormality?

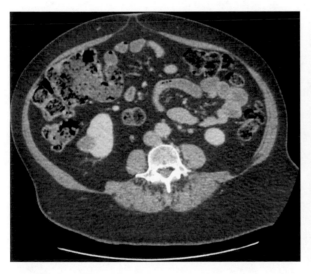

Image 1

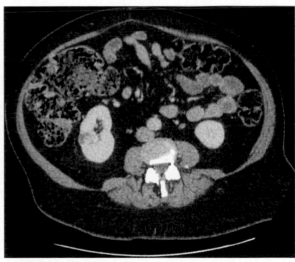

Image 2

R. Joarder et al., *Case Studies in Abdominal and Pelvic Imaging*,
DOI: 10.1007/978-0-85729-366-4_81, © Springer-Verlag London Limited 2011

Answers

1. The region is predominately low attenuation with some high attenuation flecks peripherally (Image 3) and soft tissue density, at its medial margin (Image 4). The features are those of a 'complex' renal cyst.
2. A classification of renal cysts based on their CT characteristics was suggested by Bosniak in 1986. It is used to guide management. The region shows enhancement compared to an unenhanced CT (not shown). This cyst would be classified as a type III.
3. Type III lesions are suggestive of malignancy and are generally biopsied or surgically explored.

The Bosniak classification (originally published in Radiology in 1986) attempts to separate those renal cysts requiring surgery or intervention from those that can be watched. The original categorisation was from I to IV and was subsequently revised and category II was subdivided.

The revised classification is:

I.   Simple cyst with water content, no wall thickening calcification or enhancement. They are benign.
II. Cysts containing thin septations (<1 mm), fine mural calcification or contents of increased attenuation. Category II cysts measure 3 cm or less and do not show contrast enhancement. They are benign.

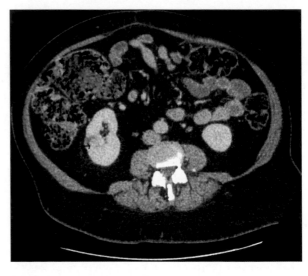

Image 4

IIF. Cysts with multiple category II features or those not fitting neatly in to category II and needing follow-up.
III. More complicated cysts with thickened wall or septae, nodular or irregular calcification or non-enhancing soft tissue. These are indeterminate lesions and, whilst they may be benign, need histological evaluation.
IV. Cysts with non-uniform or enhancing walls, wall nodularity or definite soft tissue components. These lesions are considered malignant.

> **Key Points**
>
> › Classification of renal cysts guides management.
> › Type IIF cysts require active follow-up and type III need histological evaluation.

Further Reading

Curry N, Cochran S, Bissada N (2000) Cystic Renal Masses: Accurate Bosniak Classification Requires Adequate Renal CT. AJR 175:339-342

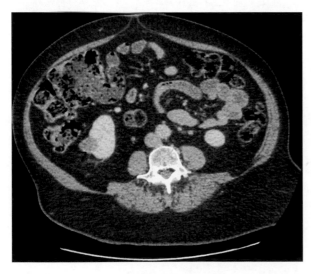

Image 3

A 40-year-old male presented with acute onset of abdominal pain, nausea, vomiting and absolute constipation. No history of abdominal surgery.

On examination his abdomen was distended but there was no peritonism. A diagnosis of small bowel obstruction was made and an MDCT of the abdomen performed (Image 1 axial and Image 2 coronal).

Questions

1. Describe the small bowel findings.
2. What is the diagnosis?

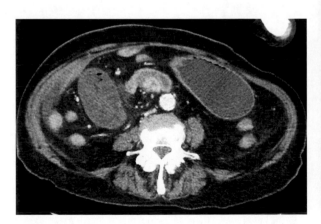

Image 1

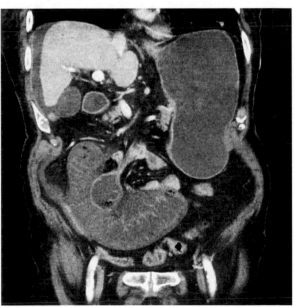

Image 2

R. Joarder et al., *Case Studies in Abdominal and Pelvic Imaging*,
DOI: 10.1007/978-0-85729-366-4_82, © Springer-Verlag London Limited 2011

Answers

1. The small bowel is distended (*long arrows* Images 3 and 4) and there is narrowing of a segment of jejunum which has twisted with its accompanying mesenteric vessels (*short arrows* Images 3 and 4) (the Whirl sign).
2. Small bowel obstruction due to small bowel volvulus.

Small bowel volvulus is a relatively uncommon cause of small bowel obstruction – it can be primary or secondary (i.e. Meckel's diverticulum or malrotation/ileosigmoid knotting). Sudden onset small bowel obstruction in the absence of previous abdominal surgery should raise the possibility of small bowel volvulus. The imaging modality of choice is CT with accuracy of 83%. MDCT enables multiplanar reconstructions to allow visualisation of the volvulus (best shown in the plane perpendicular to the plane of rotation). The point of rotation is often demonstrated with two loops of small bowel and accompanying vessels rotating around each other (the whirl sign). The loops of bowel between the two twisted loops dilate (closed loop dilation) and can necrose due to vascular compromise.

Treatment is surgical – in the absence of bowel necrosis untwisting the volvulus is usually successful; however if bowel necrosis is present bowel resection and primary anastamosis is necessary.

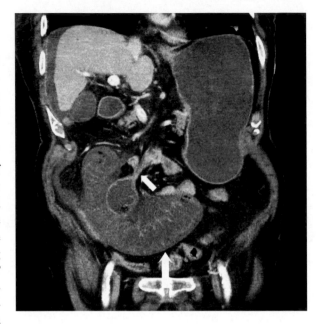

Image 4

Key Points

> Consider small bowel volvulus in sudden-onset small bowel obstruction with no history of previous abdominal surgery.
> MDCT is the best imaging modality for small bowel obstruction and demonstrates small bowel volvulus.
> MDCT signs of small bowel volvulus are the whirl sign and small bowel dilatation.

Further Reading

Ruiz-Toyar J, Morales V, Sanjuanbenito A, et al. (2009) Volvulus of the small bowel in adults. Am Surg 75(12):1179-82

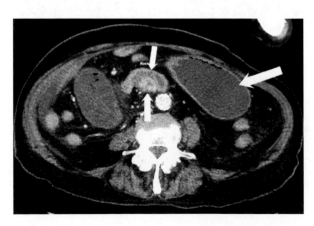

Image 3

An 82-year-old male patient with abdominal pain. Bloods revealed mildly deranged liver function tests with an obstructive pattern. US and MRCP showed intra- and extra-hepatic duct dilatation but no gallstones. An MDCT was performed to further assess the pancreas (Images 1a and b). The CT confirmed persistent mild biliary dilatation but no pancreatic mass. Blood cultures grew gram negative bacilli and a diagnosis of biliary sepsis was made. This was successfully treated with antibiotics.

Questions

1. What incidental finding is revealed on the CT scan?
2. What potential complications are associated with this abnormality?

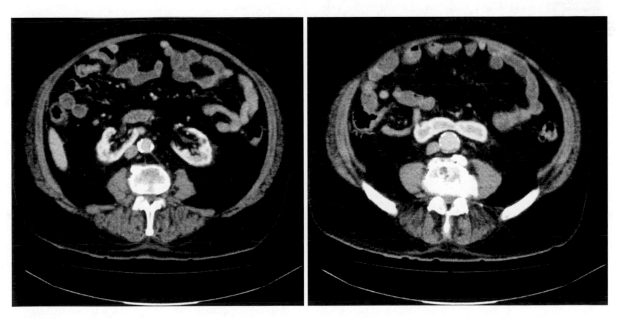

Image 1

R. Joarder et al., *Case Studies in Abdominal and Pelvic Imaging*,
DOI: 10.1007/978-0-85729-366-4_83, © Springer-Verlag London Limited 2011

Answers

1. A horseshoe kidney (Image 2).
2. Stone disease, pelviureteric junction obstruction, trauma, infections and tumours.

Horseshoe kidney is one of a group of congenital fusion anomalies where both kidneys are fused together in early embryonic life. There is a 2.3:1 male predominance, in approximately 0.25% of the population [1].

The fusion can be symmetric (midline as in this case) or asymmetric where most of the kidney lies to one side of the spine. Most (>90%) are fused at the inferior pole.

Horseshoe kidney can be associated with other congenital abnormalities in approximately a third of cases. However, around one third of patients remain asymptomatic. The most common cause for symptoms is due to urinary tract infection and stones.

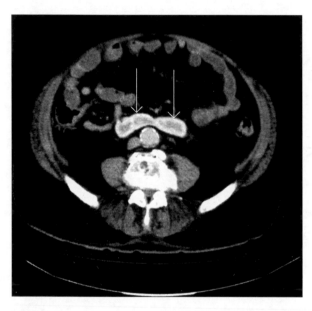

Image 2

Key Points

> One-third of horseshoe kidneys are asymptomatic and picked up incidentally.
> One-third of horseshoe kidneys are associated with other congenital abnormalities.
> Symptoms usually relate to infection or stones.

Reference

1. Weizer A.Z. et al (2003) Determining the incidence of horseshoe kidney from radiographic data at single institution. J.Urol. 170(5): 1722-6

A 30-year-old man presented to the Emergency Department with a sudden-onset severe right-sided lion pain. Urinalysis showed microscopic haematuria.

A CT scan was performed.

Questions

1. What type of scan has been performed?
2. What does the scan show?
3. What is the treatment?

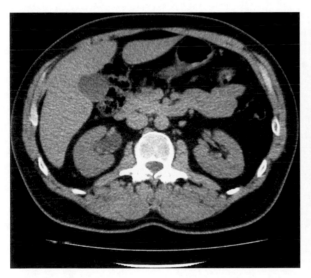

Image 1

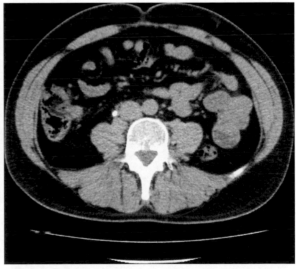

Image 2

R. Joarder et al., *Case Studies in Abdominal and Pelvic Imaging*,
DOI: 10.1007/978-0-85729-366-4_84, © Springer-Verlag London Limited 2011

Answers

1. A non-contrast CT scan of the abdomen and pelvis has been performed termed a CT KUB.
2. There is mild dilation of the right renal pelvis and right ureter (compare with the left, Image 3). There is a calcific density in the mid right ureter (Image 4). The features of a obstructing right ureteric stone.
3. A conservative approach is usually the first option. Most ureteral stones will pass spontaneously (about 70% of stones up to 5 mm). Pain relief is important with the non-steroidal agent diclofenac of particular value.

    Interventional approaches involve pharmacological active stone expulsion or active stone removal. This is most commonly used for stones greater than 7 mm, in the presence of infection, obstruction of a single kidney or bilateral obstruction. In general obstruction is relieved either by nephrostomy and stenting with later shock wave therapy or ureteroscopic removal.

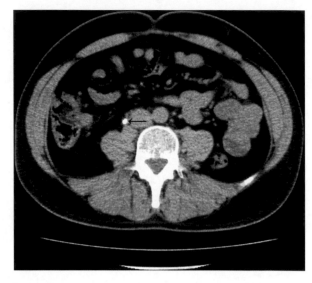

Image 4

Non-contrast MDCT has replaced intravenous urography in the diagnosis of renal or ureteric stones. Modern low dose techniques allow confident diagnosis without exposing the patient to the higher levels of radiation of a conventional CT of the abdomen and pelvis. In addition, as the whole abdomen and pelvis is visualised other alternative pathologies are often identified.

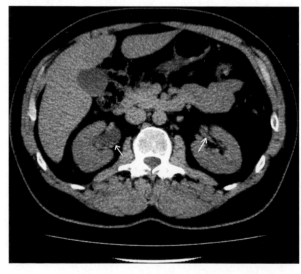

Image 3

Key Points

> Renal colic is a common presenting complaint.
> Most cases are treated conservatively.
> Non-contrast MDCT is the investigation of choice in the acute stage.

Further Reading

Poletti P, Platon A, Rutschmann O et al (2007) Low-dose versus standard-dose CT protocol in patients with clinically suspected renal colic. Am J Roentgenol 188(4):927-33

A 70-year-old patient with a history of open aortic aneurysm repair presented with haematemesis. The patient was shocked. OGD revealed a large amount of blood in the stomach and duodenum, but the cause was not demonstrated and MDCT (intravenous contrast but no oral contrast) was performed (Image 1 axial and Image 2 sagittal).

Questions

1. What is the round contrast containing structure posteriorly?
2. What is the round contrast containing structure anterior to the rounded area identified in question 1?
3. What is the liner track between these two areas of opacification?
4. What is the diagnosis?
5. What are the treatment options?

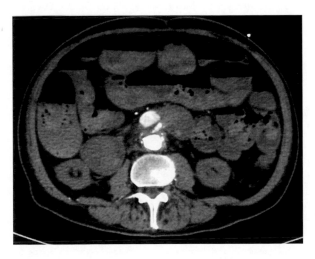

Image 1

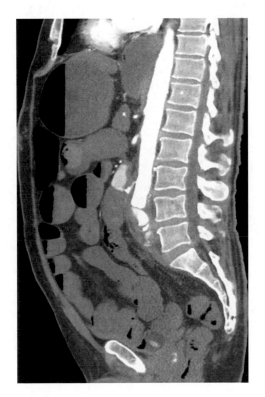

Image 2

R. Joarder et al., *Case Studies in Abdominal and Pelvic Imaging*,
DOI: 10.1007/978-0-85729-366-4_85, © Springer-Verlag London Limited 2011

257

Answers

1. The aorta (or more accurately the superior anastamosis of the aortic graft to native aorta) (*long arrow* Images 3 and 4).
2. The duodenum (*short arrow* Images 3 and 4).
3. Aortoduodenal fistula (*medium arrow* Images 3 and 4).
4. Secondary aortodoudenal fistula – a complication of the previous AAA repair.
5. Surgical or endovascular repair.

If a patient who has previously had an aortic aneurysm repair (open or endovascular stent graft) presents with GI bleeding, a secondary aortoenteric fistula should be considered (and probably assumed unless proven otherwise). The upper anastamosis of the graft to the aorta lies very close to the third part of the duodenum. If there is communication between the two then catastrophic GI bleeding can result although there is often a preceding herald bleed. It is thought that low grade infection of the anastamosis plays a significant aetiological role and some patients present with sepsis.

OGD may reveal a large amount of blood in the upper GI tract. MDCT is often diagnostic if the patient is bleeding (as in this case) but can be normal if not bleeding at the time of scanning.

Conservative treatment is almost universally fatal. Surgery (graft excision with axillobifemoral graft or

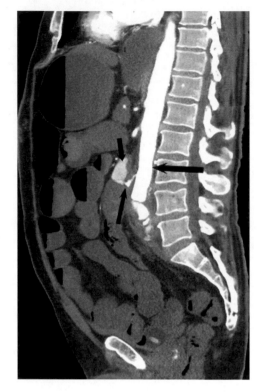

Image 4

graft replacement) or endovascular repair with a stent graft is required. Patients who present with shock have a poor prognosis.

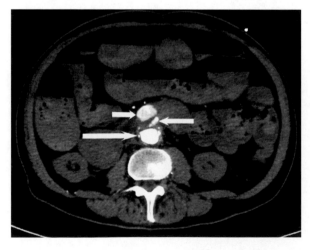

Image 3

Key Points

> If patients with previous AAA repair present with GI bleeding, assume an aortodoudenal fistula until proven otherwise.
> MDCT is diagnostic if bleeding at the time of scanning.
> Surgery or endovascular repair is required.

Further Reading

Armstrong PA, Back PR, Wilson JS, et al. (2005) Improved outcomes in the recent management of secondary aortoenteric fistula. J Vasc Surg 42(4):606-6

A 61-year-old male patient with a long history of cardiac failure and ventricular arrhythmias presented to the chest physicians with a persistent cough. On examination he was found to have basal crackles, and pulmonary function tests showed a slightly reduced transfer factor. A high resolution CT (HRCT) of the thorax, which is performed without intravenous contrast, was therefore arranged (Images 1a and b). The HRCT showed normal lung parenchyma but revealed an abnormality within the upper abdomen.

Questions

1. What do Images 1a and b show?
2. What is the likely cause?
3. What test would you recommend and why?

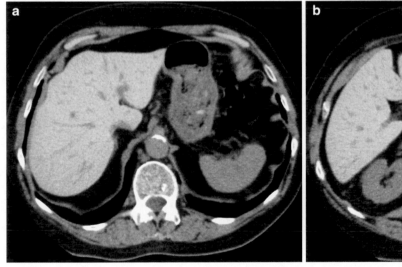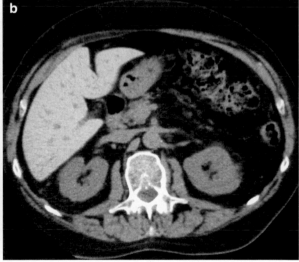

Image 1

R. Joarder et al., *Case Studies in Abdominal and Pelvic Imaging*, DOI: 10.1007/978-0-85729-366-4_86, © Springer-Verlag London Limited 2011

Answers

1. There is a general diffuse increased attenuation of the liver (*long arrow* Image 2) compared with the spleen (*short arrow* Image 2).
2. Amiodarone deposition within the liver.
3. Liver function tests (LFTs), as a small proportion may have a significant hepatitis.

Amiodarone is an iodinated compound used to treat refractory ventricular arrhythmias. In addition to being a potential cause of pulmonary toxicity, it is known to accumulate within the liver and can cause in these patients a phospholipidosis within the hepatocytes [1]. CT shows a significant increased attenuation of the liver in patients who have Amiodarone accumulation here.

In one series [2], 25% of 104 patients taking Amiodarone had an asymptomatic rise in aminotransferase and 3% had symptomatic hepatitis. Serial liver function tests are recommended by the manufacturer; however, levels of Amiodarone may persist within the liver for weeks or months after stopping the drug. Clearly, risks of hepatotoxicity should be weighed against cardiac risk when considering stopping Amiodarone.

Other causes of increased hepatic density on CT include haemochromatosis, haemosiderosis, other drugs such as gold and thallium.

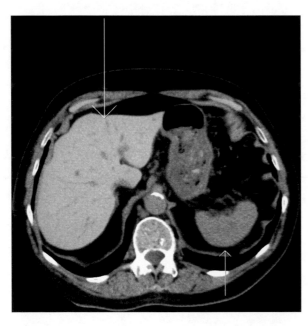

Image 2

Key Points

> Increased density of the liver relative to the spleen particularly on an unenhanced scan in a patient with a significant cardiac history is suggestive of Amiodarone deposition.

> Amiodarone accumulation only causes abnormal LFTs in a small proportion of patients and only a proportion of these have symptomatic hepatitis.

> The LFTs should be checked if a high density liver is seen at CT.

References

1. Goldman IS et al (1985). Increased hepatic density and phospholipidosis due to Amiodarone. AJR 144(3): 541-546
2. Lewis J.H. et al (1989). Amiodarone hepatotoxicity: Prevalence and clinicopathologic correlations among 104 patients. Hepatology, 9(5): 679-685

A 70-year-old man presented to the Emergency Department with a short history of colicky abdominal pain and vomiting. On examination his bowel sounds were increased. An AXR was performed followed by an MDCT.

Questions

1. What does the AXR show?
2. What does the CT show?
3. What is the diagnosis?

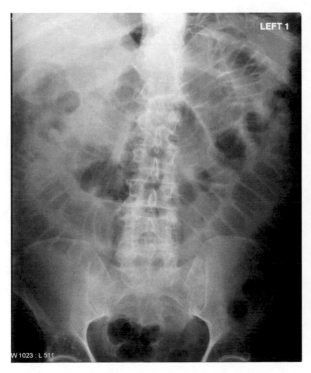

Image 1

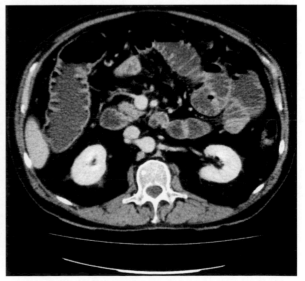

Image 2

Image 3

R. Joarder et al., *Case Studies in Abdominal and Pelvic Imaging*,
DOI: 10.1007/978-0-85729-366-4_87, © Springer-Verlag London Limited 2011

Answers

1. The abdominal X-ray shows multiple dilated loops of small bowel (Image 4 *arrows*) and proximal large bowel. There is no evidence of intra-abdominal free gas.
2. The CT confirms the presence of small bowel dilatation with dilatation of the caecum and ascending colon. The more distal large bowel is collapsed. There is soft tissue thickening of the wall of the proximal transverse colon which is not distended (Image 5 *arrow*).
3. The diagnosis is of bowel obstruction caused by a carcinoma of the transverse colon. In this case there is mild dilatation of the large bowel proximal to the lesion with marked dilatation of the small bowel.

Small bowel obstruction is considered when bowel diameter exceeds 2.5 cm on plain film. Small bowel obstruction (SBO) can be divided into high and low grade. High grade is considered when small bowel dimensions average 36 mm and exceed 50% of the

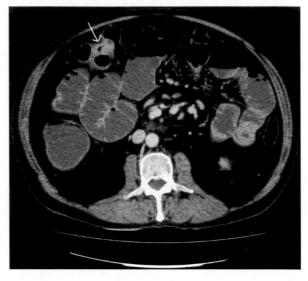

Image 5

calibre of the largest visible loops of colon. Small bowel loops can be differentiated from large bowel by having lines that traverse their whole width (valvae coniventes) as opposed to the partial haustral pattern of large bowel.

MDCT is useful in the investigation of SBO. It is a quick examination and oral contrast is not generally required as the retained fluid acts as negative contrast agent. The whole bowel is demonstrated allowing easier analysis. The cause and site of obstruction is also more likely to be demonstrated which is important in directing management.

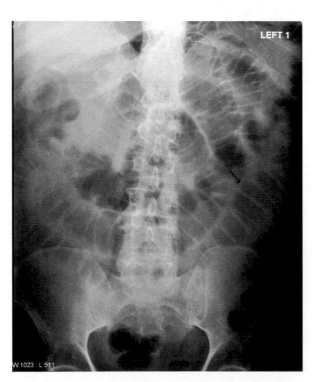

Image 4

> ### Key Points
>
> › Small bowel dilation may result from obstructing abnormalities within the large bowel if the ileocaecal valve is incompetent.
> › MDCT is the investigation of choice.

Further Reading

Silva A, Pimenta M, Guimaraes L (2009) Small bowel obstruction: what to look for. Radiographics 29 (2): 423-39

A 50-year-old male with a history of excess alcohol consumption presented with several weeks of central abdominal pain. The amylase was normal but the white count, ESR and CRP were elevated. MDCT (Image 1) and US were performed. Several months later the patient re-presented with abdominal distension and vomiting. Another MDCT was performed (Image 2).

Questions

1. Comment on the pancreas in Image 1.
2. Comment on the pancreas in Image 2.
3. What is the diagnosis?
4. What therapy should be considered?

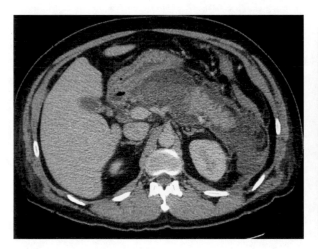

Image 1

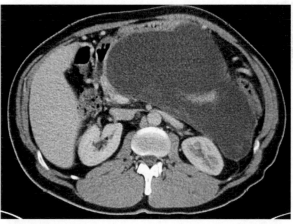

Image 2

R. Joarder et al., *Case Studies in Abdominal and Pelvic Imaging*,
DOI: 10.1007/978-0-85729-366-4_88, © Springer-Verlag London Limited 2011

Answers

1. The pancreatic head, tail and neck are swollen, non-enhancing with a fairly well-defined margin (*short arrows* Image 3). The pancreatic body is enhancing normally (*long arrow* Image 3).
2. The pancreatic body is still enhancing but is now surrounded by a large, encapsulated fluid collection (*arrow* Image 4).
3. Acute severe pancreatitis complicated by pseudocyst formation.
4. Endoscopic drainage of the pseudocyst (stent placed from stomach to pseudocyst).

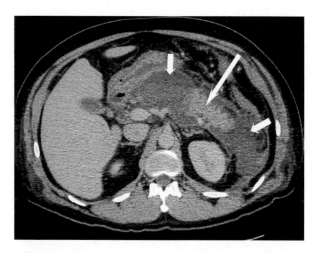

Image 3

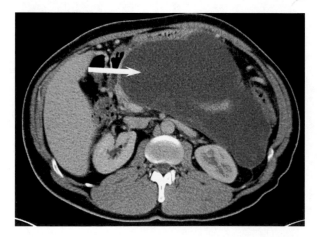

Image 4

Pancreatitis is most often mild and self-limiting. However severe pancreatitis often requires extensive imaging. US is often performed in the first 24 h to identify patients with gallstones who may benefit from early ERCP and sphincterotomy. Ultrasound does not reliably visualise the pancreas. The gold standard is MDCT. This is usually performed between 4 and 7 days after onset of symptoms (although can be earlier if there is doubt over the diagnosis). MDCT reliably assesses the degree of necrosis which is the main determinant of prognosis [1]. The CT grading of pancreatitis is more accurate than clinical or biochemical grading in predicting morbidity and mortality [2]. CT can also identify most of the many and varied complications of pancreatitis. In this case the patient had evidence of necrosis of more than 50% of the pancreas and a fluid collection putting them into the worst prognostic group with over 90% chance of a complication and 17% mortality [1]. The initial image shows an acute extra-pancreatic fluid collection which matured into a pseudocyst (as shown by the presence of a capsule around the collection). Pseudocysts often resolve spontaneously but may need aspiration/drainage if large, symptomatic or infected. This is often performed endoscopically to allow drainage into the stomach (potentially avoiding a cutaneous pancreatic fistula from direct percutaneous drainage).

Key Points

> MDCT is gold standard for imaging acute severe pancreatitis.
> MDCT accurately quantifies degree of necrosis which accurately predicts the course of the disease.

References

1. Balthazar EJ, Robinson DJ, Megibow AJ. (1990) Acute pancreatitis: value of CT in establishing prognosis. Radiology 174:331-336
2. Van den Biezenbos AR, Krupty PM, Bosscha K. (1998) Added value of CT criteria compared with the clinical SAP score in patients with acute pancreatitis. Abdom Imaging 23:622-626

A 41-year-old male presented with a long history of frequent loose stools and more recent weight loss. Sigmoidoscopy revealed an impassable tight stricture in the sigmoid colon.

Questions

1. What type of study has been performed in Image 1?
2. What does it show?
3. What does Image 2 show?
4. What type of study has been performed in Images 3a–c?
5. What does it show?
6. What is the most likely diagnosis?

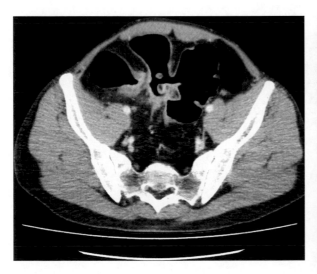

Image 1

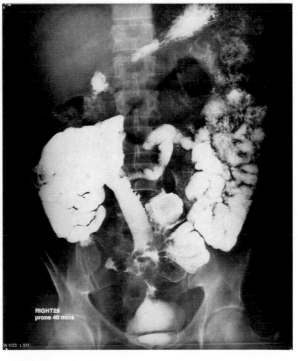

Image 2

R. Joarder et al., *Case Studies in Abdominal and Pelvic Imaging*, DOI: 10.1007/978-0-85729-366-4_89, © Springer-Verlag London Limited 2011

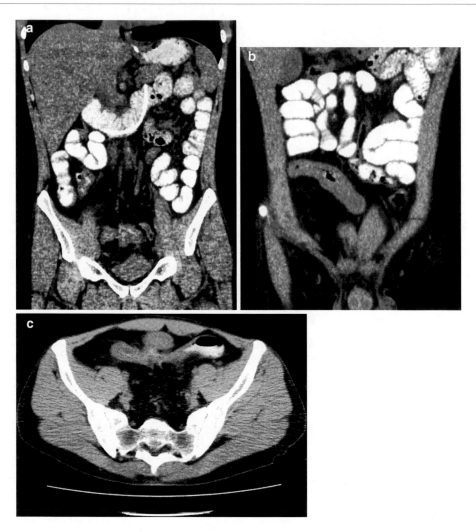

Image 3

Answers

1. CT colonography.
2. A fistulous connection between the sigmoid colon and distal ileum.
3. The barium follow through confirms the fistula (*oblique arrow* Image 4) with early contrast seen within the rectum (*horizontal arrow* Image 4).
4. CT enteroclysis with a naso-jejunal tube in situ (*horizontal arrow* Image 5).
5. It shows thickened matted loops of distal ileum and confirms the fistula between the distal ileum and the sigmoid (Images 6a and b).
6. Crohn's disease.

CT enteroclysis is a technique which has improved the ability to visualise small bowel pathology but is generally reserved for problem solving in complex cases of Crohn's disease, low grade small bowel obstruction and small bowel tumours. This can help particularly for surgical planning. The technique involves the placing of a naso-jejunal tube (by an endoscopist in our

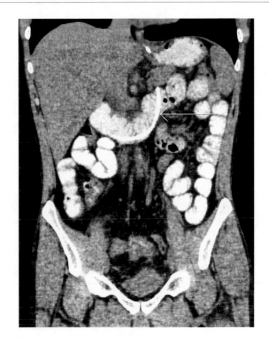

Image 5

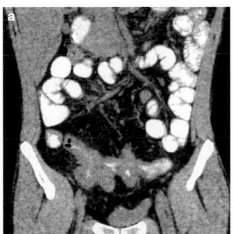

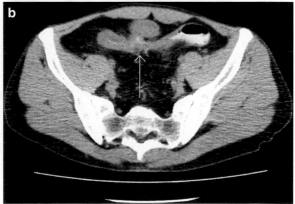

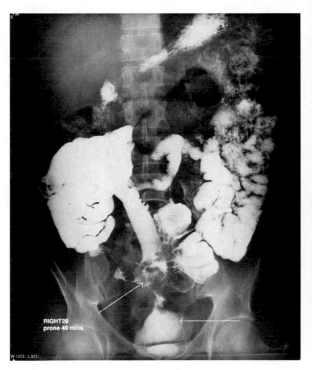

Image 4

Image 6

institution) and administering 2L of positive contrast directly into the small bowel.

MDCT allows mutiplanar reconstructions which are particularly useful when examining bowel loops and their relation to adjacent tissues. Image 6a is a coronal CT reconstruction which shows the thickened small bowel loops. Image 6b shows the fistulous connection between the small and large bowel (*arrows*). We tend to perform the study without intravenous (IV) contrast as we are using positive small bowel contrast; however, an alternative technique is to administer water to the small bowel and give IV contrast.

Key Points

> CT enteroclysis is generally reserved for problem solving in cases of small bowel pathology.
> 2L of contrast instilled via a naso-jejunal tube.
> Improves distension of small bowel loops as contrast instilled quicker than achieved by drinking.
> Allows assessment of small bowel pathology in relation to other tissues.

Further Reading

Schmidt S et al (2005) CT enteroclysis; technique and clinical applications. European Radiology. 16(3):648-660

A 50-year-old female was seen in A/E with acute abdominal pain.

Her erect chest X-ray was unremarkable. Her full blood count showed a low HB of 8 g/dL, with raised white count (25) and platelet count (690).

MDCT of her abdomen and pelvis was performed.

Questions

1. What abnormalities does the CT show?
2. What acute event has occurred?
3. What may be the underlying cause?
4. If the patient survives, what long-term problems may occur?

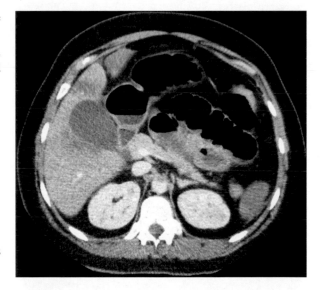

Image 2

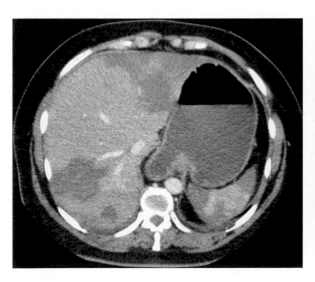

Image 1

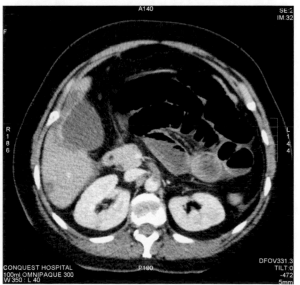

Image 3

R. Joarder et al., *Case Studies in Abdominal and Pelvic Imaging*,
DOI: 10.1007/978-0-85729-366-4_90, © Springer-Verlag London Limited 2011

Answers

1. There is patchy altered (non) enhancement in the liver and spleen (Image 4). There is small bowel dilatation with a hazy alteration of the attenuation of the mesenteric fat. There is enhancement of the duodenum and very proximal jejunum but not of more distal small bowel.

   The superior mesenteric arty (SMA) is not enhancing and there is low attenuation at the origin of the artery from the aorta (Image 5 *black arrow*). There is further low attenuation at the origin of the coeliac axis (CA).

2. There is acute occlusion of the SMA with partial occlusion of the CA. This is resulting in small bowel ischaemia and ultimately necrosis. There is also infarction of the spleen and arterial ischaemia of the liver. Flow is seen in the portal vein although the return from the spleen and SMV is much reduced.

3. There may be a thrombophilic tendency from the raised platelet count, and the patient was thought to have essential thrombocythaemia.

4. The patient did survive but underwent multiple operations for resection of necrotic small bowel. She was left with only 15 cm. Loss of small bowel causes problems with nutrition and malabsorption (short bowel syndrome). Total parenteral nutrition may be required.

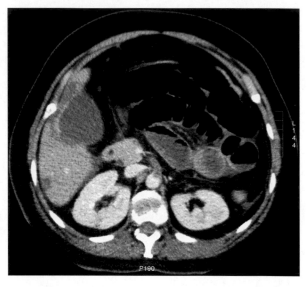

Image 5

Short bowel syndrome is a long term malabsorption state that results from extensive resection of the small bowel. Features include nutrient electrolyte and vitamin deficiency, diarrhoea, dysmotility and bowel dilatation. It has been a frequent complication of multiple resections in patients with Crohn's disease. With improvement in treatment both medical and surgical for the latter condition it is now more frequently a complication of vascular disorders (infraction) in adults or congenital abnormalities in children. The remaining bowel does undergo a process termed adaptation which can be encouraged by medical treatment. If nutrition cannot be maintained orally, parenteral support will be required long term. This has its own inherent risks, e.g., cholestatic liver disease.

Some surgical options are available including intestinal transplantation although these are currently used as a last resort.

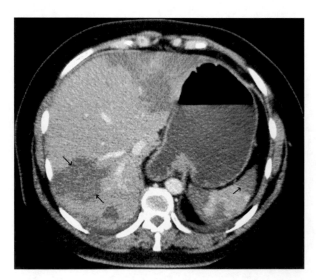

Image 4

> **Key Points**
>
> › Mesenteric ischaemia from vascular occlusion may present without prior symptoms and is often fatal.
> › Multiple small bowel resections can lead to a malabsorptive state.

Further Readings

Keller J, Panter H, Layer P. Management of the short bowel syndrome after extensive small bowel resection. Best Pract Res Clin Gastroenterol. 2004 Oct;18(5):977-92

Misiakos EP, Macheras A, Kapetanakis T, Liakakos T. Short bowel syndrome: current medical and surgical trends. J Clin Gastroenterol. 2007 Jan;41(1):5-18

An 83-year-old female, previously fit and well with a long history of smoking, presented with several months of generalised abdominal pain after eating. She reported weight loss of 2 stones over the same period.

Blood tests and US and OGD were normal.

A CT angiogram was performed (Image 1, sagittal CT through origin of SMA: Image 2, axial CT through origin of SMA; Image 3, axial CT through coeliac axis).

Questions

1. Comment on the coelic axis and SMA.
2. What is the diagnosis?

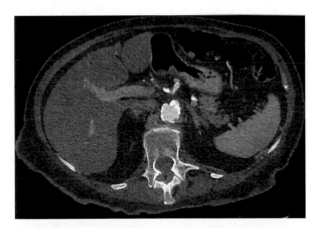

Image 2

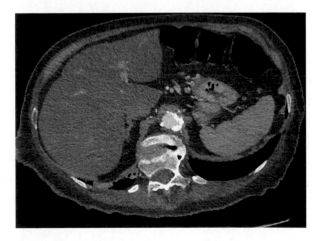

Image 3

Image 1

R. Joarder et al., *Case Studies in Abdominal and Pelvic Imaging*,
DOI: 10.1007/978-0-85729-366-4_91, © Springer-Verlag London Limited 2011

Answers

1. Severe, heavily calcified stenoses are demonstrated at the origins of both the coeliac and SMA (*arrows* – Images 4, 5 and 6).
2. Mesenteric angina due to atheromatous stenosis of the mesenteric arteries.

The diagnosis of mesenteric angina secondary to severe atheromatous stenosis of the coeliac and SMA was made and the patient referred to the Interventional Radiology department for endovascular intervention.

The intra-arterial angiogram confirmed a tight stenosis at the origin of the SMA (*arrow* – Image 7). This was crossed with a guide wire (*long arrow* on stenosis and *short arrow* on guide wire – Image 8). A balloon-expandable stent was placed across the SMA stenosis and dilated to 6 mm (*arrow* – Image 9).

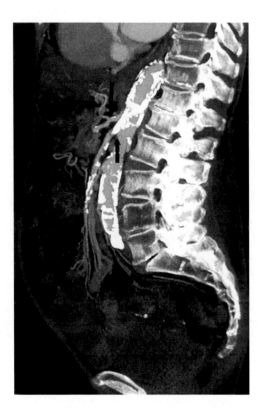

Image 4

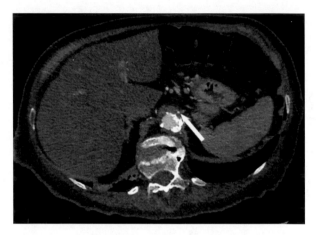

Image 6

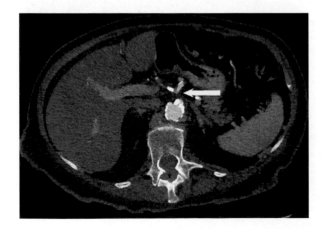

Image 5

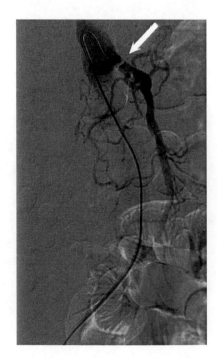

Image 7

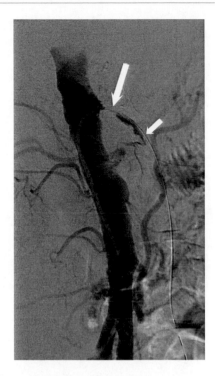

Image 8

The post-stent insertion angiogram (Image 10) showed abolition of the SMA stenosis (*long arrow*) with some non-occlusive thrombus in the main SMA trunk (*short arrow*). The patient's abdominal pain resolved and the lost weight was regained.

Mesenteric angina is an uncommon cause of post-prandial abdominal pain and weight loss. The diagnosis is often delayed. The diagnosis should be borne in mind, particularly in elderly patients with risk factors for atherosclerosis and evidence of ischaemia in other systems. The diagnosis can be made by non-invasive imaging including Doppler US (although this requires considerable expertise), CTA and MRA.

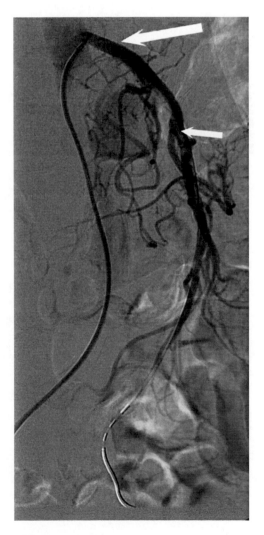

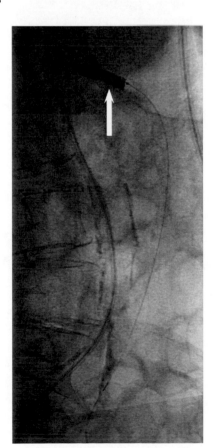

Image 9   **Image 10**

The condition usually has a prolonged course which results in the formation of multiple collateral channels. Thus for symptoms to occur significant disease of two of the three (SMA, IMA, coeliac) splanchnic arteries is necessary.

Although surgical bypass has, until recently, been the treatment of choice, less invasive endovascular options, including stent insertion, are now preferred.

Early intervention is often advised for symptom relief and prevention of progression to acute, life threatening ischaemia causing bowel infarction. Intervention in asymptomatic patients is more controversial. Although there is a significant risk of becoming symptomatic which is said to carry a 40% mortality. However intervention has its own morbidity and mortality.

Key Points

> Mesenteric angina should be considered in elderly patients with post-prandial pain, weight loss and atherosclerosis.
> CTA is diagnostic – severe disease of at least two of the three splanchnic arteries is required to give symptoms.
> Treatment of choice is endovascular stent insertion.

Further Reading

Sreenarasimhaiah J (2005) Chronic Mesenteric Ischemia. Best Pract Res Clin Gastroenterol 19(2):283-295

A 17-year-old female presented with a month's history of worsening perianal pain. An MDCT of the pelvis (Images 1a and b) was performed. A course of antibiotics was prescribed and the patient was then followed up after a period of 6 weeks with MRI (images 2a–c and 3a and b).

Questions

1. What do Images 1a and b show?
2. What do Images 2a–c show?
3. What is the low signal structure annotated with the arrow in Images 3a and b?
4. What condition should be excluded in this patient?

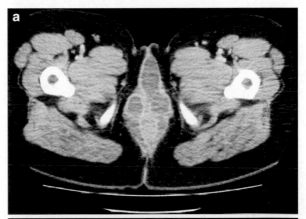
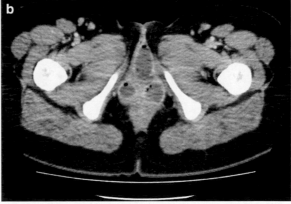

Image 1

R. Joarder et al., *Case Studies in Abdominal and Pelvic Imaging*,
DOI: 10.1007/978-0-85729-366-4_92, © Springer-Verlag London Limited 2011

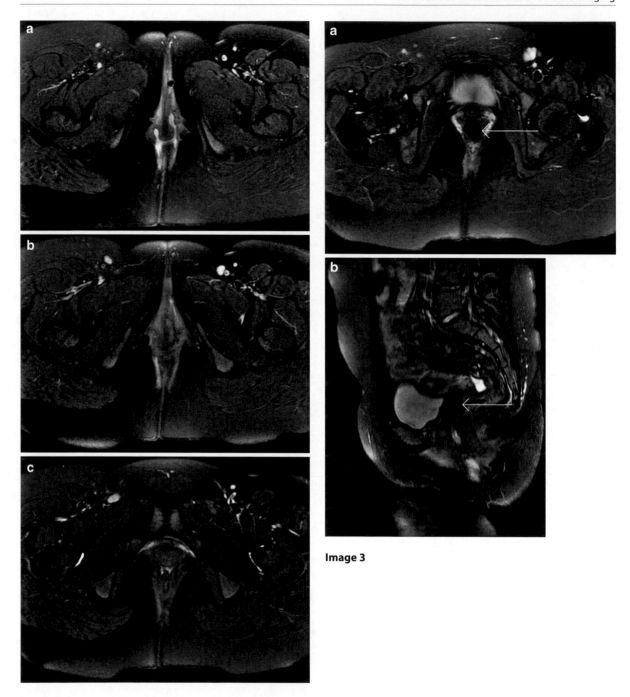

Image 2

Image 3

Answers

1. Images 1a and b show an extensive perineal abscess extending along both sides of the anal canal and vagina anteriorly into the vulval tissues. Air is noted within the abscess.

2. The MRI shows a reduction in size of the abscess but delineates its path more clearly. It has an 'H' shaped configuration extending from both buttocks close to the natal cleft to run anteriorly and connect anterior to the rectum and posterior to the vagina but does not involve the rectum or anal sphincters (*arrows* Images 4a and b). The left branch of the 'H' runs anteriorly to abut but not involve the urethra (*arrow* Image 4c). It is intersphincteric and is confined by the external sphincter and does not cross either this or the internal sphincter. It also remains below the levators and does not involve the ischiorectal fossae. It is therefore a grade 2 intersphincteric fistula with a secondary fistulous track [1].

3. The *arrow* in Image 3 points to a tampon within the vagina.

4. Crohn's disease.

MRI is the imaging modality of choice for assessing perianal fistulae and abscesses. The track of a fistula can be delineated and its relation to the internal and external anal sphincters, the levators and ischeorectal fossae. The fistula is then graded as from 1 to 4 according to the involvement of these features. The possible involvement of other structures such as the vagina and urethra can also be determined. These factors are essential for operative planning.

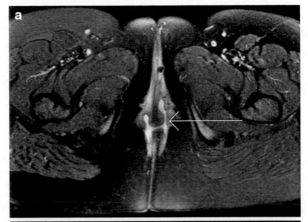
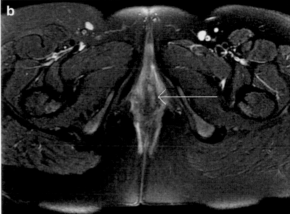
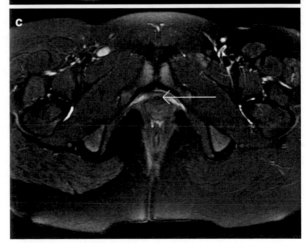

Image 4

Key Points

> MRI accurately delineates the track of perianal fistula.

> It is important to determine whether the track is inter- or transphincteric, single or complex, whether it involves the ischeorectal fossae and whether it crosses the levators.

Reference

1. Morris J et al (2000) MR imaging classification of perianal fistulas and its implications for patient management. Radiographics 20:623-635

A 75-year-old male underwent abdominal imaging for investigation of weight loss and anaemia.

Questions

1. What abnormality does the scan show?
2. What complications may occur?
3. What are the treatment options?

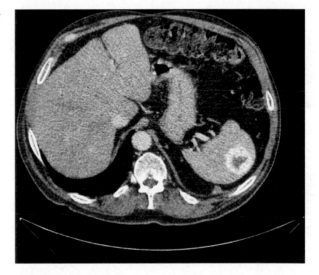

Image 1

Answers

1. There is a mixed attenuation lesion in the spleen. This shows central low (Image 2 *white arrow*) and peripheral slightly nodular high attenuation (*black arrow*). The features are consistent with a haemangioma.
2. Lesions that are large or multiple and occupy the whole spleen may rupture and bleed.
3. Most are incidental and require no treatment, although splenectomy may be required.

Splenic haemangiomas are the most common primary splenic tumour with a quoted incidence at autopsy of 0.03–14%. The majority are found incidentally or at post-mortem. They are derived from sinusoidal epithelium, and being slow growing are more likely to present in adults.

Imaging features reflect those of hepatic haemangioma with peripheral nodular enhancement in the arterial phase followed by delayed fill on venous and later phase imaging.

US typically shows a well-marginated highly reflective lesion which may be avascular on colour Doppler. Microbubble contrast shows enhancement and larger lesions may show centripetal enhancement. On MRI the lesions are typically high on T2 with centripetal and persistent enhancement on delayed images.

Spontaneous rupture is reported in up to 25%. Splenectomy is a common prophylactic treatment. Observational follow-up of certain sized lesions may be preferred.

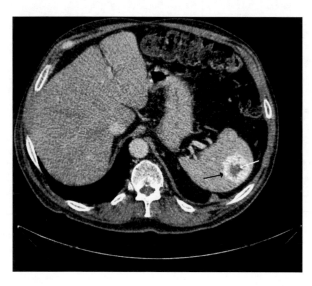

Image 2

> ### Key Points
>
> › splenic haemangiomas are usually coincidental findings.
> › Rupture is a recognised complication.

Further Reading

Wilcox T, Speer R, Schlinkert R, Sarr M. (2007) Hemangioma of the spleen: Presentation, diagnosis, and management. J Gastrointestinal Surgery vol 4 (6) 611-613

A 55-year-old female presenting with non-specific central abdominal pain and vomiting was referred for MDCT of the abdomen (Image 1 axial CT).

Questions

1. Describe the appearance of the mesenteric fat.
2. What diagnoses should be considered?

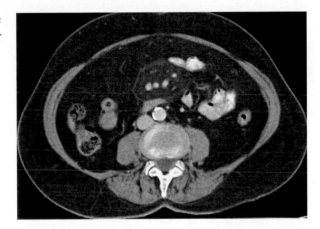

Image 1

R. Joarder et al., *Case Studies in Abdominal and Pelvic Imaging*,
DOI: 10.1007/978-0-85729-366-4_94, © Springer-Verlag London Limited 2011

Answers

1. The central mesenteric fat, around the mesenteric vessels (*long arrow* Image 2), is hyper-attenuating and has a subtle pseudo-capsule (*short arrows* Image 2).
2. Sclerosing mesenteritis (SM), but there is a wide differential (see text below).

'Misty mesentery' is the term used to describe hyper-attenuating mesenteric fat seen on CT and raises the possibility of 'sclerosing mesenteritis' (SM). SM is a non-specific, benign inflammatory process affecting the adipose tissue of the mesentery of unknown cause. It is known by many other names including mesenteric panniculitis, Weber-Christian disease, to name but two.

The clinical features are non-specific and can include abdominal pain, vomiting, weight loss and rectal bleeding. An abdominal mass can be palpitated in 50% of patients. SM generally has a self-limiting course.

CT demonstrates the fat in the affected area to have attenuation values of between –40 and –60 Hounsfield units (as opposed to –100 to –160 normally). The mesenteric vessels are encased but not displaced; there are soft tissues nodules (usually less than 5 mm) in 80% and a thin (less than 3 mm) pseudo-capsule in 50%.

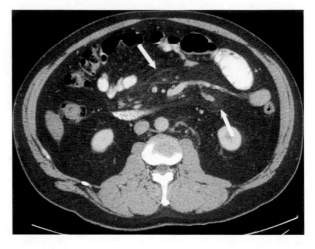

Image 3

'Misty mesentery' can occur in many other conditions including malignancy (such as NHL (*arrows* Image 3), carcinoid and desmoids), inflammation such as pancreatitis and mesenteric oedema from any cause, i.e. cirrhosis, heart failure.

Because of this differential diagnosis biopsy is sometimes performed unless the CT features are typical of SM – see above.

Key Points

> Misty mesentry is hyper-attenuating fat seen on CT.
> There are several causes ranging from self-limiting SM to NHL.

Further Readings

Joerger M, Nueslli DF, Henz F, et al. (2008) CT-diagnosed mesenteric alterations with non-Hodgkin's lymphoma: a population based study. Onkologie; 31(10):514-9

Wat SY, Harish S, Winterbottom A, et al. (2006) The CT appearances of sclerosing mesenteritis and associated diseases. Clin Radiol 61(12):652-8

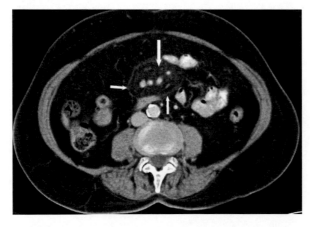

Image 2

A 73-year-old female smoker presented with a 2-week history of left-sided abdominal pain and 1-day history of fresh rectal bleeding. Past history included cardiac failure for which she was followed up by the cardiologists. There was no significant gastro-intestinal history. On examination she was tender in the left upper quadrant. She had a minimally raised WBC and was passing fresh blood and mucus. An AXR (Image 1) and a CT of the abdomen and pelvis (Images 2a–d) were performed.

Questions

1. What does Image 1 show?
2. What do Images 2a–d show?
3. What is the most likely diagnosis?

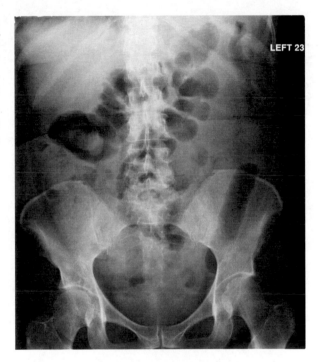

Image 1

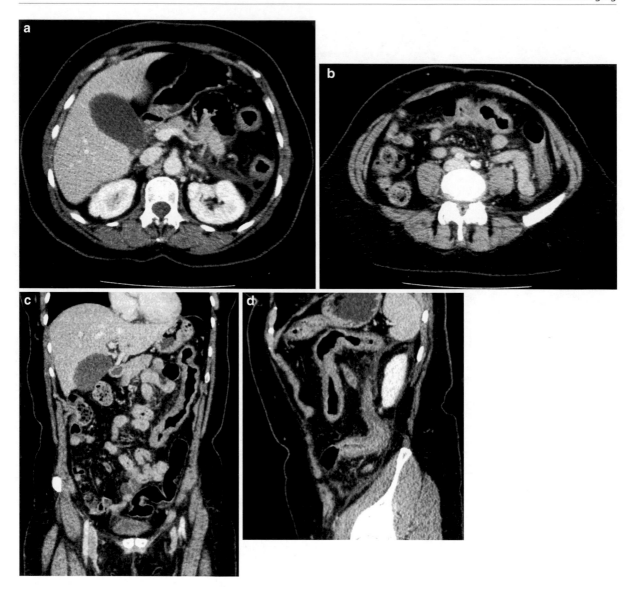

Image 2

Answers

1. Narrowing and oedema of the distal transverse (*vertical arrow* Image 3) and proximal two thirds of the descending colon (*horizontal arrows* Image 3).
2. The CT scan images show a long, thick-walled stricture involving the distal half of the transverse colon to continue into and involve the proximal two thirds of the descending colon (Images 4a–d).
3. Ischaemic colitis.

Ischaemic colitis is a condition found predominantly in elderly patients and is linked to various predisposing factors including atherosclerotic heart disease, cardiac and aortic surgery, myocardial infarction and hypotensive episodes. It is a form of non-occlusive ischaemic disease affecting most commonly the segment of bowel at the watershed between the territories supplied by the superior and inferior mesenteric arteries near the splenic flexure and the watershed between the inferior mesenteric artery and hypovascular supply at the rectosigmoid junction.

In the acute phase there is haemorrhage, oedema and necrosis of the bowel mucosa which can be self-limiting and reversible. If there is necrosis of the muscle layer this can lead to stricture formation (as in this case) but also severe sepsis and occasionally perforation.

CT findings therefore are of the range of appearances. In this case a long, thick-walled stricture involving the splenic flexure was seen. Stricture lengths can vary. Other reported cases have also seen air within the bowel wall [1], oedema and marked pericolic streakiness.

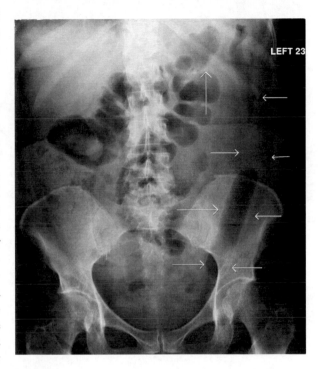

Image 3

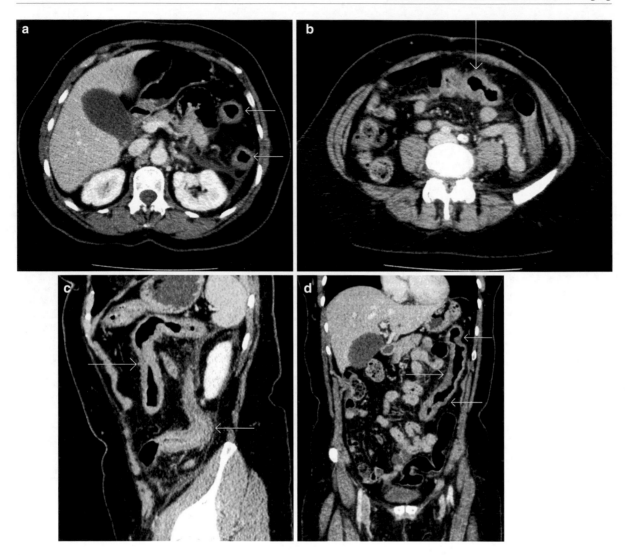

Image 4

Key Points

> If a stricture is seen at the splenic flexure consider ischaemic colitis.

> Ischaemic colitis should particularly be considered with long strictures (carcinomas are usually shorter).

> This form of ischaemia is non-occlusive.

Reference

1. Balthazar EJ et al (1999) Ischemic colitis: CT evaluation of 54 patients. Radiology 211:381-388

A 78-year-old woman with a history of diverticular disease was seen in the out patient clinic. She gave a history of noticing blood on toilet paper. Sigmoidoscopy in out patients was unsuccessful due to pain.

CT colonography was requested.

Questions

1. What do Images 1 and 2 show?
2. What does Image 3 show?

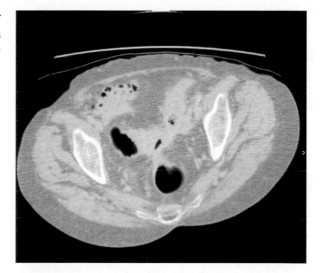

Image 2

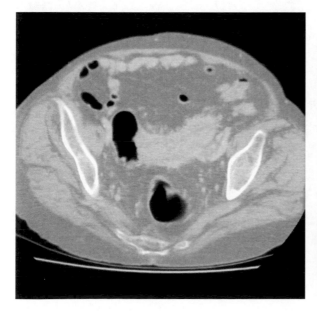

Image 1

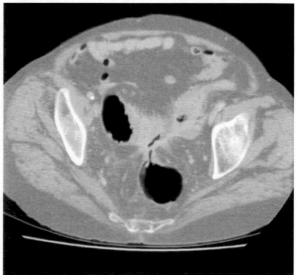

Image 3

R. Joarder et al., *Case Studies in Abdominal and Pelvic Imaging*,
DOI: 10.1007/978-0-85729-366-4_96, © Springer-Verlag London Limited 2011

Answers

1. There is a section of bowel in the sigmoid region that does not distend on either the supine (Image 4) or prone (Image 5) views. There is a little pericolic stranding. Given that the study is a VC with rectal insufflation, a fixed lack of distension is consistent with stricture formation.
2. There is a low attenuation linear region passing from the area of apparent stricture formation into the rectum (Image 6). This would be consistent with a fistulous connection.

Stricture formation occurs in both benign and malignant diseases.

    Benign causes in adults include:

    Inflammatory bowel disease (Crohn's/ulcerative colitis)

    Diverticulitis

    Infections, e.g., histoplasmosis

    Endometriosis

    Post-treatment, e.g., anastomotic or post-radiotherapy

Diverticular disease is common. Complications of diverticular disease include haemorrhage, perforation, abscess formation, stricture formation and inflammatory fistulation. Diverticular strictures are usually relatively long (>6 cm) and of relatively smooth appearance. The features are however not absolute and histological examination post-resection is essential.

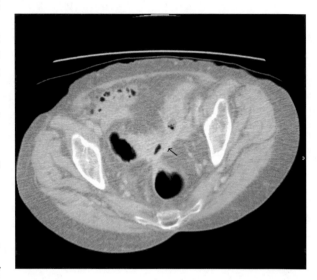

Image 5

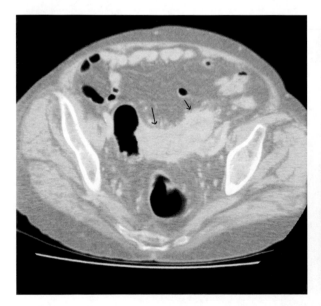

Image 4

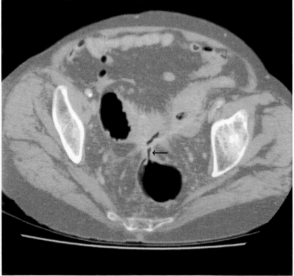

Image 6

Key Points

> CT colography is a useful investigation after failed sigmoidoscopy/colonoscopy.

> Stricture formation is common in diverticular disease and may be associated with fistula formation.

Further Reading

Yucel C, Lev-Toaff A Moussa N, Durrani H (2008) CT colonography for incomplete or contraindicated optical colonoscopy in older patients. Am J Roentgenol 190(1):145-50

Case 97

A 34-year-old female with a 6-week history of endo-carditis, proven on blood cultures and echocardiography, presented with sudden onset severe abdominal pain and shock. An urgent MDCT was performed (Images 1 and 2 contrast-enhanced axial images).

Questions

1. Describe the abnormal findings.
2. What is the likely explanation?

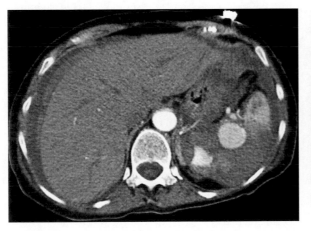

Image 1

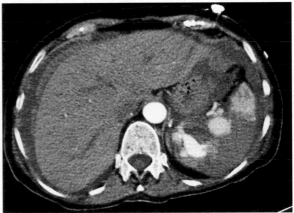

Image 2

R. Joarder et al., *Case Studies in Abdominal and Pelvic Imaging*,
DOI: 10.1007/978-0-85729-366-4_97, © Springer-Verlag London Limited 2011

Answers

1. There is a well-defined rounded high attenuation opacity in the left upper quadrant (*long arrows* Image 3 and 4). Just medial to this is a more irregular area of higher attenuation (*star* Images 3 and 4). There is free fluid of two densities around the liver and in the left upper quadrant (*short arrows* Images 3 and 4).
2. This is most likely to be a ruptured mycotic aneurysm of the splenic artery (*long arrow* Images 3 and 4) with extravasation of contrast (*star* Images 3 and 4) and blood in the peritoneum (*short arrows* Images 3 and 4).

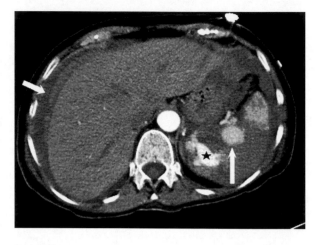

Image 4

The ruptured splenic artery aneurysm was assumed to have been mycotic in origin in view of proven endocarditis. The mycotic aneurysm was asymptomatic until rupture, which resulted in catastrophic intra-abdominal haemorrhage. The contrast extravasation is due to active bleeding and indicates the need for urgent intervention. In this case urgent surgery with

ligation of the splenic artery and splenectomy was performed. Alternatively it could have been treated endovascularly in the angiography suite by embolisation (a technique which is useful in splenic trauma) which gives rapid control of haemorrhage and preservation of the spleen.

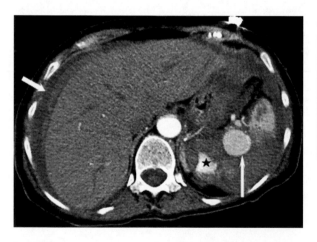

Image 3

Key Points

> Mycotic aneurysms can complicate endocarditis.
> Mycotic aneurysms can present with life-threatening haemorrhage.
> IR is an effective way of treating mycotic aneurysms – both ruptured and unruptured.

A 54-year-old female patient presented with a 5-week history of recurrent rectal bleeding. A barium enema was performed (Images 1a and b).

Questions

1. What do Images 1a and b show?
2. What is the diagnosis?

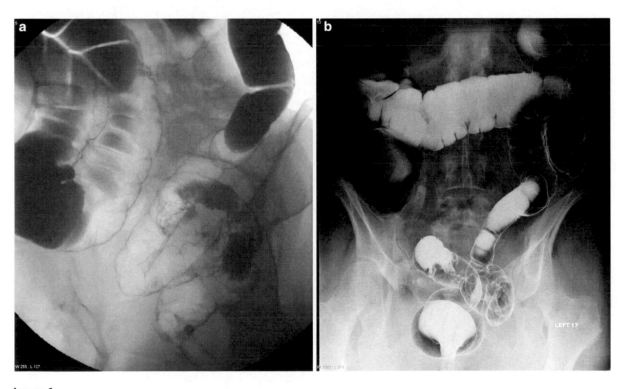

Image 1

R. Joarder et al., *Case Studies in Abdominal and Pelvic Imaging*, DOI: 10.1007/978-0-85729-366-4_98, © Springer-Verlag London Limited 2011

Answers

1. There is an apple core lesion within the rectum (Images 2a and b).
2. Rectal carcinoma.

Whilst more and more centres are performing CT colonography instead of barium enemas, they have not become obsolete. This is due to resource and capacity issues that most hospitals share. There is still a significant number of barium enemas performed.

The lesion within the rectum is partly obscured by overlapping bowel, but if the study is examined carefully it is easily visible (Images 2a and b).

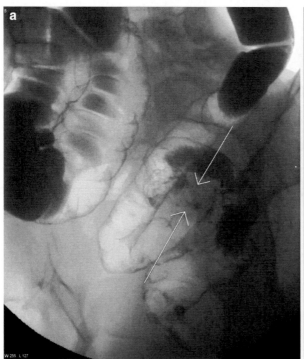
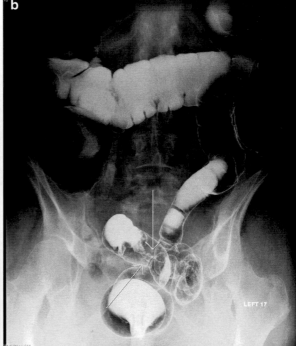

Image 2

A 79-year-old male was investigated for a single episode of painless macroscopic haematuria. There was no significant post-medical history. Flexible cystoscopy was normal. Ultrasound showed prominence of the right pelvicalyceal system with no other abnormality and a normal left system.

MDCT is requested.

Questions

1. What is the differential diagnosis for the PC system distension seen on US and what is the most likely diagnosis?
2. What do Images 1 and 2 show?
3. What does Image 3 show?

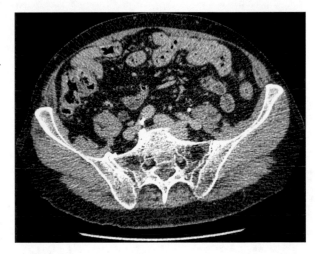

Image 2

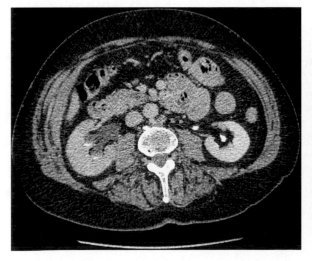

Image 1

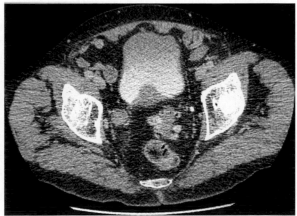

Image 3

R. Joarder et al., *Case Studies in Abdominal and Pelvic Imaging*,
DOI: 10.1007/978-0-85729-366-4_99, © Springer-Verlag London Limited 2011

Answers

1. There is evidence of right-sided renal collecting system dilatation with a normal bladder. This implies a ureteric abnormality or abnormality at the vesico–ureteric junction not visible from inside.

   Causes can be divided as follows:

   Intraluminal, e.g., tumours, stones, strictures, fungus balls.

   Intramural, e.g., mega ureter.

   Extramural, e.g., retroperitoneal fibrosis, compression by adjacent malignancy (e.g., prostate or ovarian) or lymph nodes.

   In this case, given the history, malignant compression is the most likely either intrinsic or extrinsic.

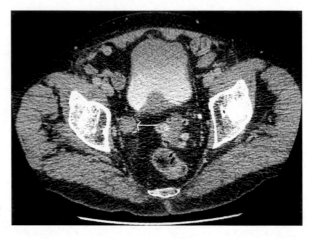

Image 6

2. There is pelvicalyceal system distension (Image 4) and ureteric distension (Image 5). There is also poor contrast filling of the right ureter as a result of reduced renal function caused by the obstruction.
3. There is an enhancing soft tissue density in the distal ureter consistent with an urothelial tumour (Image 6).

A transitional cell carcinoma is the most likely tumour of the lower ureter as the transitional cell urothelium lines the tract from bladder to renal pelvis.

Relief of obstruction can be achieved by various routes. A percutaneous nephrostomy will give initial decompression if renal function is compromised. If excision is not an option, longer term patency can be achieved with ante- or retro-grade stent insertion.

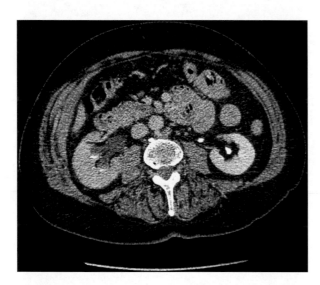

Image 4

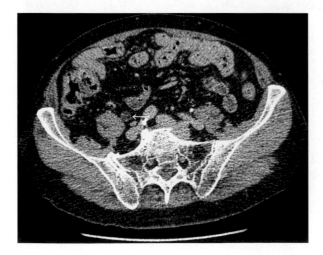

Image 5

Key Points

> Full assessment of the upper renal tracts is required in patients with unexplained haematuria.

> Ureteric obstruction can be relieved percutaneously via nephrostomy or endoscopically via the bladder.

Further Reading

Liastikos E, Kamabatidis D, Katsanos K et al (2009) Ureteral metal stents: 10-year experience with malignant ureteral obstruction treatment. J Urol 182(6):2613-7

A 76-year-old lady presented to the orthopaedic team with a 1-month history of bilateral leg weakness and some loss of bladder and bowel control. A thoracolumbar MRI scan revealed a focal mass within the 7th thoracic vertebra which was causing mild cord compression and was suspicious for a bony metastasis. An MDCT of the thorax, abdomen and pelvis was performed to search for a primary lesion as she had no other symptoms (Images 1–4).

Questions

1. What do Images 1–4 show?
2. What is the likely diagnosis?
3. What is the main differential diagnosis?
4. What features help you determine the most likely pathology?

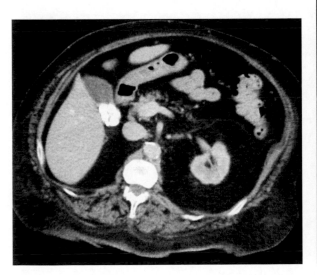

Image 1

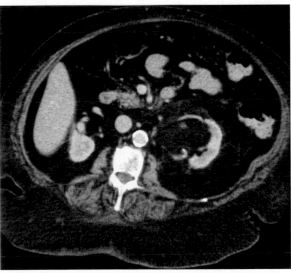

Image 2

R. Joarder et al., *Case Studies in Abdominal and Pelvic Imaging*,
DOI: 10.1007/978-0-85729-366-4_100, © Springer-Verlag London Limited 2011

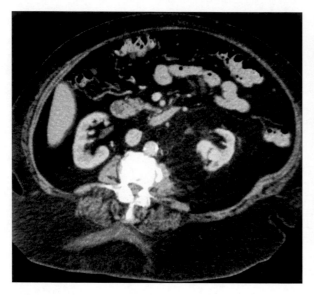

Image 3

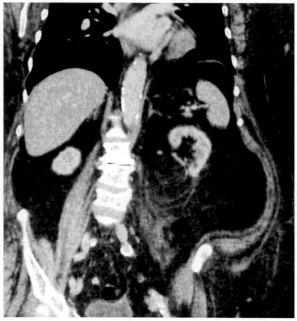

Image 4

Answers

1. A large fatty mass which is engulfing (Image 5) and displacing (Image 6) the left kidney laterally.
2. A perirenal liposarcoma.
3. A renal angiomyolipoma.
4. Renal parenchymal defects and enlarged vessels favour a diagnosis of angiomyolipoma; these are not evident here. The smooth compression of the kidney and the extension of fatty soft tissue beyond the perirenal space (Image 7) favour the diagnosis of a perirenal liposarcoma which this turned out to be.

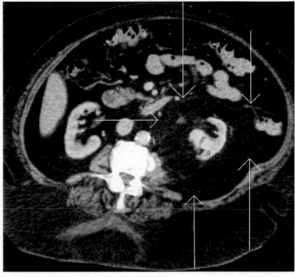

Image 7

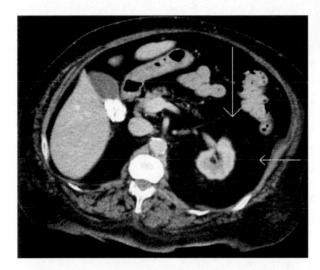

Image 5

Both the fatty perirenal mass and the thoracic vertebral metastasis were biopsied. The histology from both confirmed a liposarcoma. Renal angiomyolipomas can be large and exophytic and can appear radiolologically similar to well-differentiated perirenal liposarcomas. However, the presence of renal parenchymal defects and enlarged vessels are more in favour of a renal angiomyolipoma [1]. Also the extension of the fatty mass beyond the perirenal space favours a perirenal liposarcoma.

Key Points

> Main differential is renal angiomyolipoma.
> Renal parenchymal defects and enlarged vessels favour angiomyolipoma.
> Extension beyond peri renal fat favours perirenal liposarcoma.

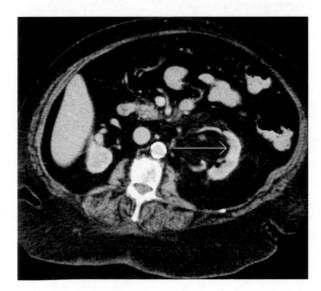

Image 6

Reference

1. Israel GM, Bosniak MA, et al. (2002) CT differentiation of large exophytic renal angiomyolipomas and perirenal liposarcoma. AJR 179:769-773